Nurse Dorothea presents Managing Anger Instead of Letting Anger Manage You

Authored by Michael Dow, RN, MS, MHA, MSM

Illustrations by Lindsay Roberts, M.Ed, BFA

Nurse Dorothea presents Managing Anger Instead of Letting Anger Manage You

Copyright © 2025 by Dow Creative Enterprises, LLC

All rights reserved

First Edition

ISBN 979-8-9905577-3-4

Printed by Lulu

Published by Dow Creative Enterprises®

Dow Creative Enterprises, LLC
PO Box 15357
Tucson, AZ 85708

Library of Congress Control Number: 2025900628

Dow Creative Enterprises® is a federally registered trademark with the United States Patent and Trademark Office.

Nurse Dorothea® is a federally registered trademark with the United States Patent and Trademark Office.

Help Civilization Reach Its Potential® is a federally registered trademark with the United States Patent and Trademark Office.

Table of Contents

Title	Page Number
Dedication	vi
Part 1	1
Part 2	89
Part 3	171
References	268
About the Illustrator	271
About the Author	273
Other Books by DCE	275

Dedication

The Nurse Dorothea book series is dedicated to Dorothea Dix. Her work in the 1800s helped people with mental illness live a more dignified life. She spent decades lobbying government officials to create state hospitals for the mentally ill. One person can make a difference.

Michael

Part 1

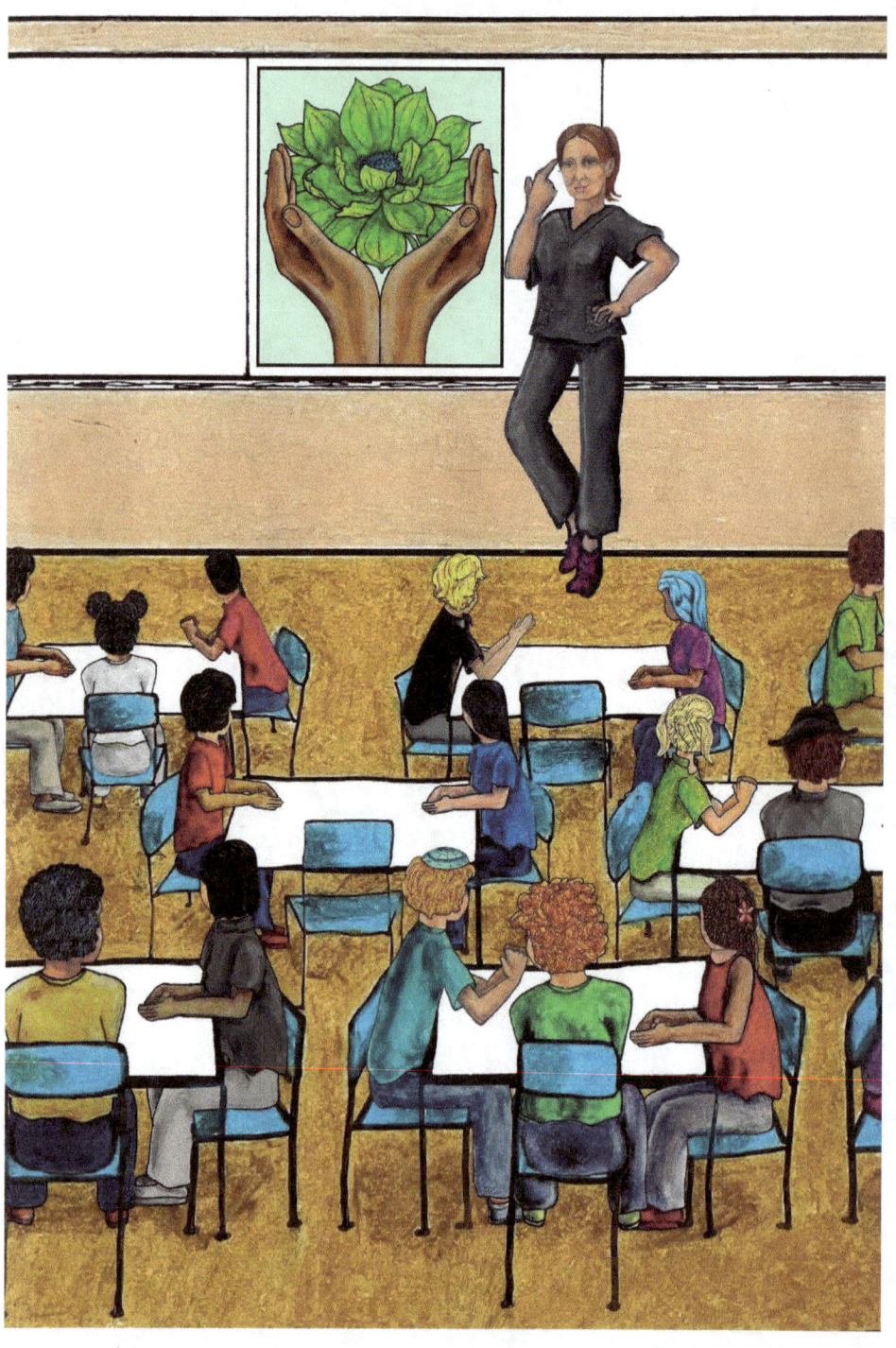

"Hi everyone. My name is Nurse Dorothea. Thank you for coming to the after-school club on mental health. I hope to provide you with some tools to manage your emotions and navigate life's challenges. Mental health is complicated because there are so many things that can affect it. This class was created to show that it's ok to talk about your mental health with others as well as give you ideas to improve your mental health."

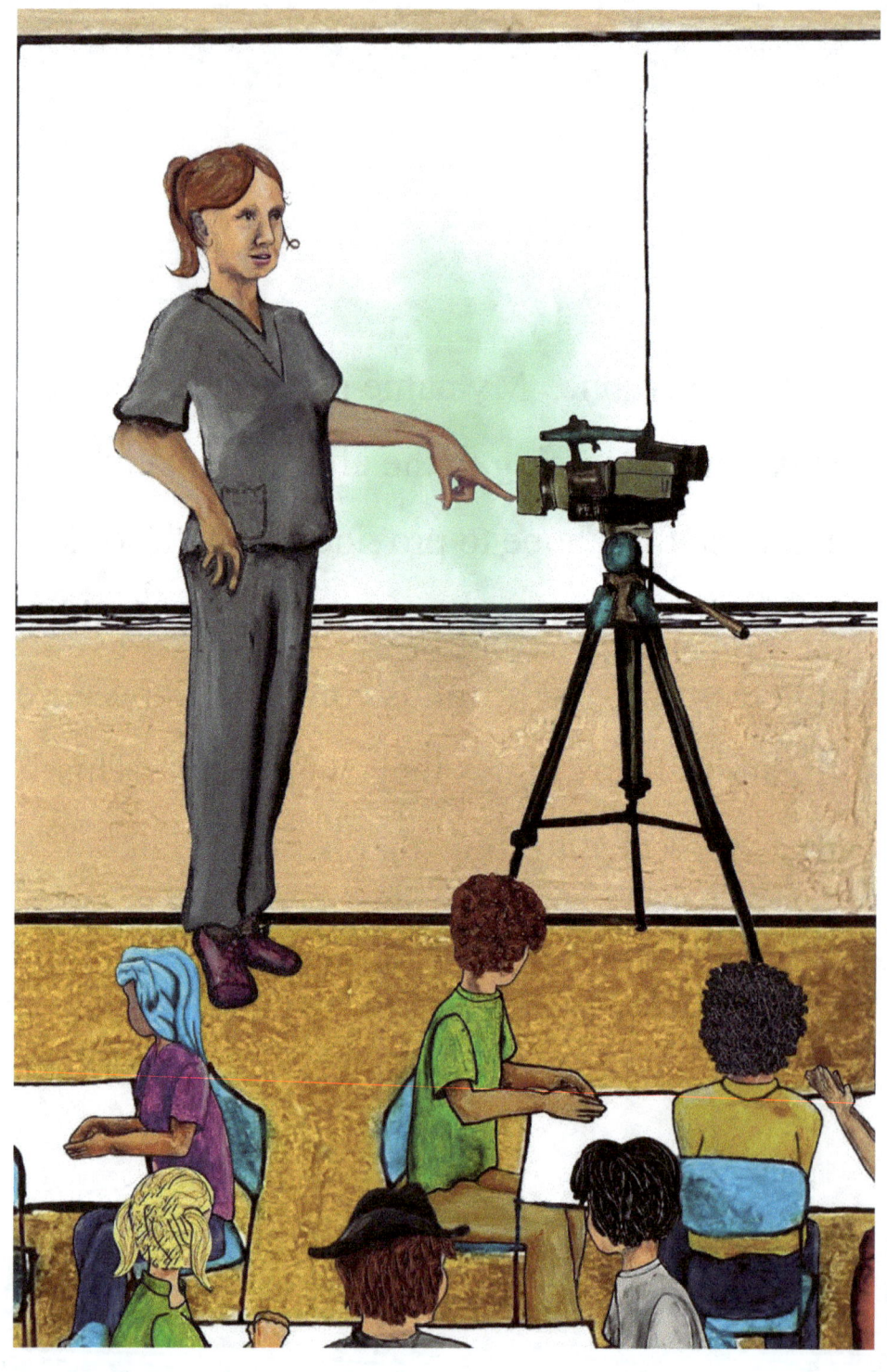

"We will be recording this session. People in the future will get to experience the same things you will today. Sometimes, I will speak to people watching this show or reading the future book about the class. This is an interactive class, and I want you all to ask questions as you have them. We will stop sometimes and discuss things with each other. If you are watching the show or reading the book, then I want YOU all to also discuss the questions and topics with those in the room. This book is an experience, and you will only get the full experience by talking with others. Please take breaks from the show as you need to, since this will be a long discussion."

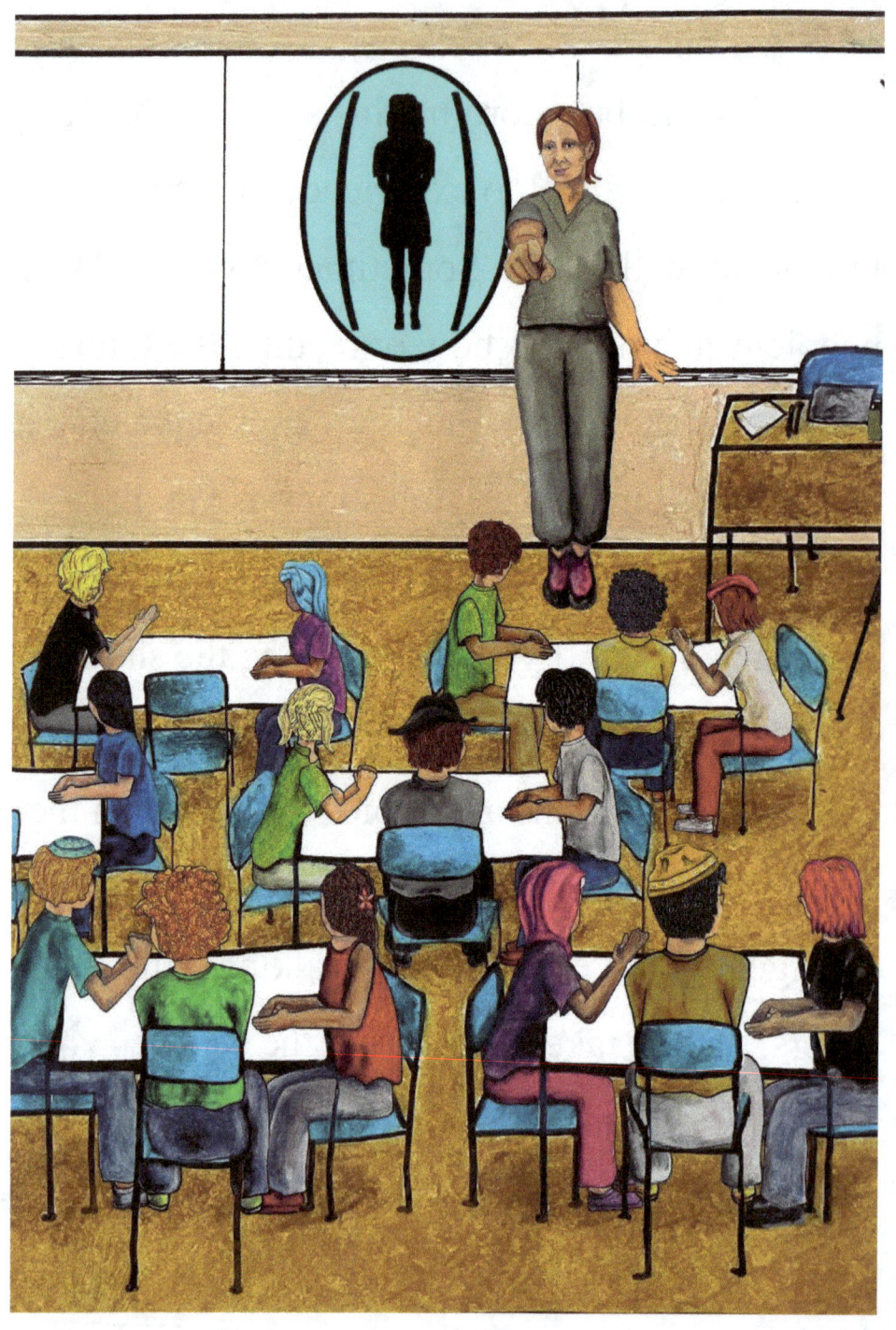

"If you are watching the show or reading this book alone, that is ok. Please take the time right now to get out a journal. I want those doing this class by themselves to write down responses to questions that I will ask, so that you participate like all the others. Sometimes, we need to address some mental health issues alone, so that is why it is ok to do this class by yourself. We are on a journey that is ultimately our own, but it is always nice to have people alongside us to help us in the bad times and share our joy in the good times."

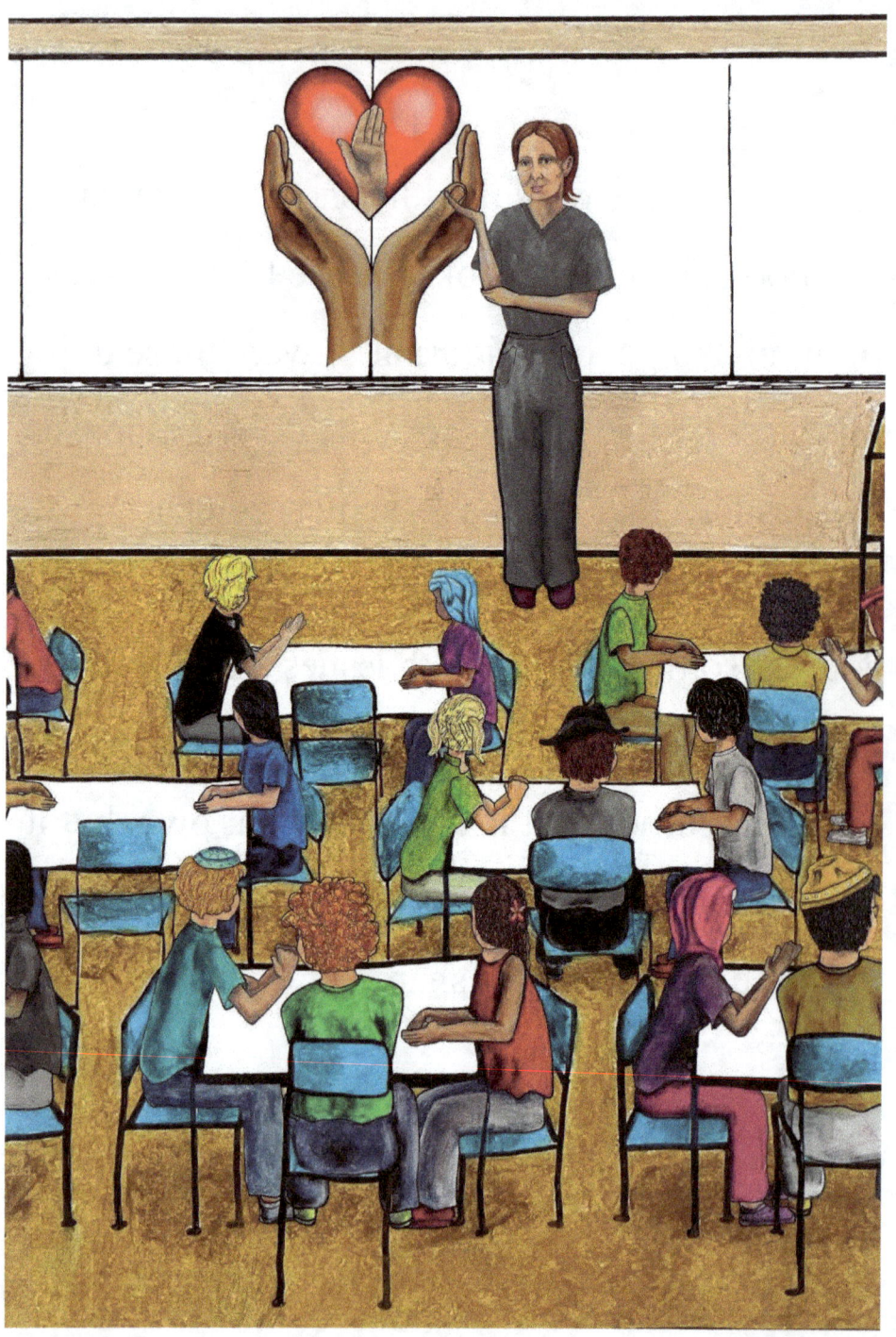

"The main rule for the class is to respect others. If someone has a question, we are to be quiet and let them speak. Raise your hand if you have a question, and I will call on you. Respecting everyone is important since we can learn from everyone. To start the class, I'd like to mention that every person is one life event away from having a mental health challenge. Some people manage life events better than others, and one negative event for one person may cause depression and anxiety. For another person, it may only cause mild frustration, because each person has different knowledge, skills, and abilities. This class is meant to help us have some common basic info."

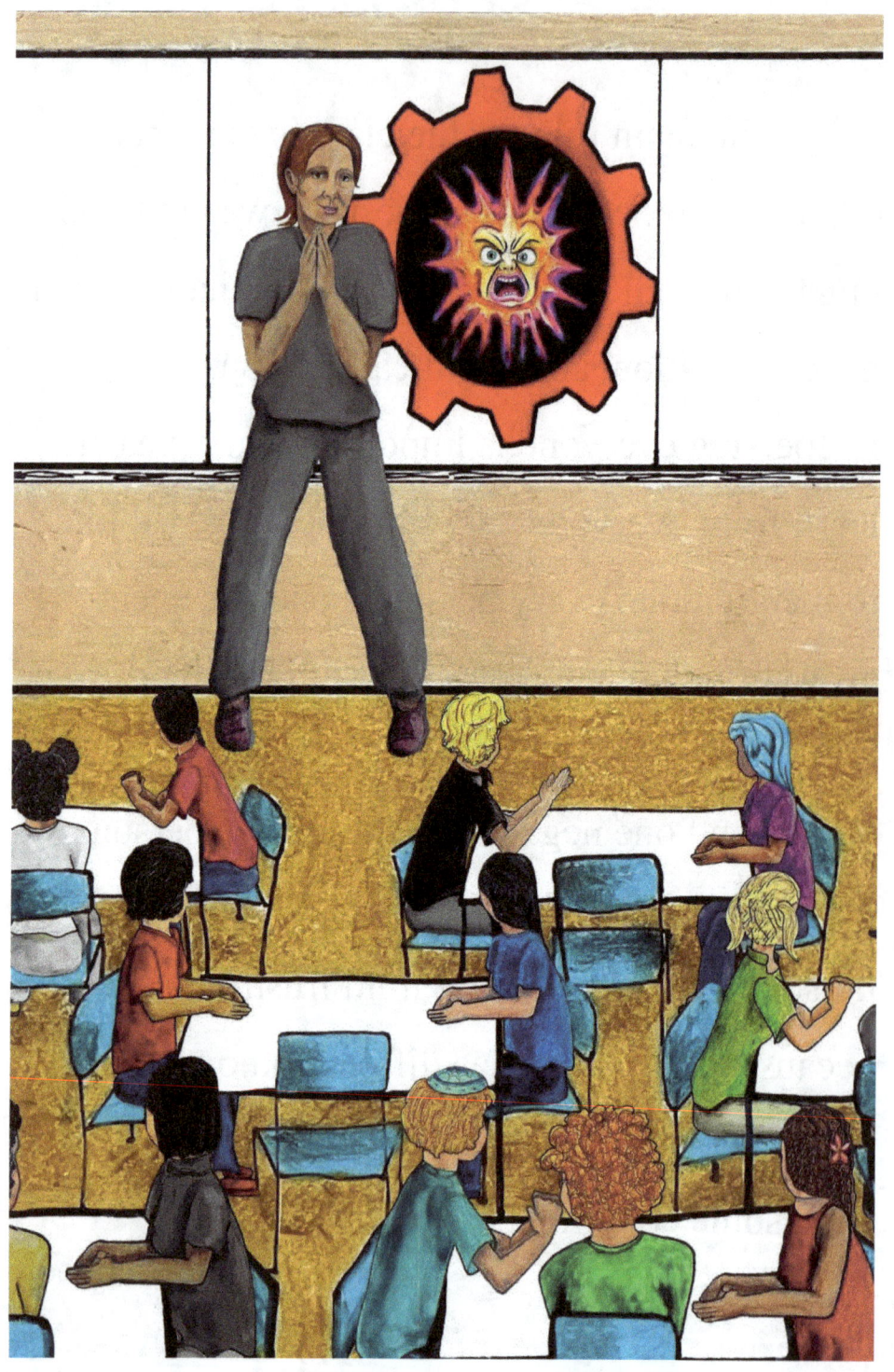

"The topic for this class is anger and learning to manage it. The American Psychological Association says anger is "an emotional state that varies in intensity from mild irritation to intense fury and rage." *Merriam-Webster* defines anger as "a strong feeling of displeasure and usually of antagonism." Rage is defined by *Merriam-Webster* as "violent and uncontrolled anger." *Cambridge Dictionary* defines anger as "a strong feeling that makes you want to hurt someone or be unpleasant because of something unfair or unkind that has happened." Dictionary.com defines anger management as "a psychotherapeutic process or program for controlling anger and preventing its destructive manifestations."

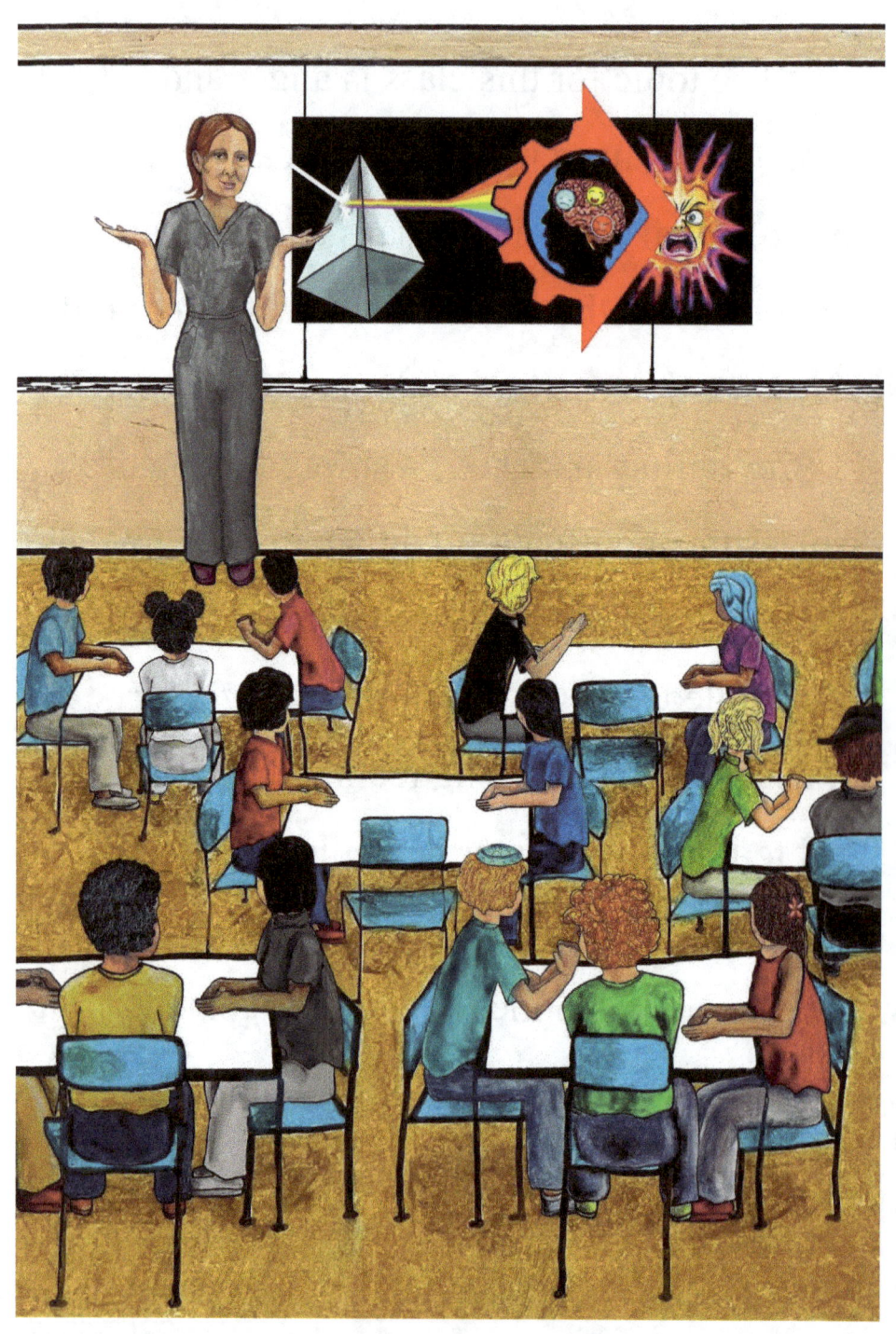

"Anger can be seen on a spectrum of natural emotions. It takes emotional courage to face your anger and learn to manage it. Anger can be triggered by external events such as a traffic jam or a person doing or saying something. Anger can also be caused by internal events such as remembering traumatic events. Different emotions can lead to anger like grief and depression. Some people have anger associated with their mood disorders, but just because you have anger does not mean you have a mental illness. We all need to find productive and safe ways to manage our anger. Managing anger is important since anger can lead us to do things or say things that we may regret. Some people do things out of anger that they regret for the rest of their lives, affecting mental well-being."

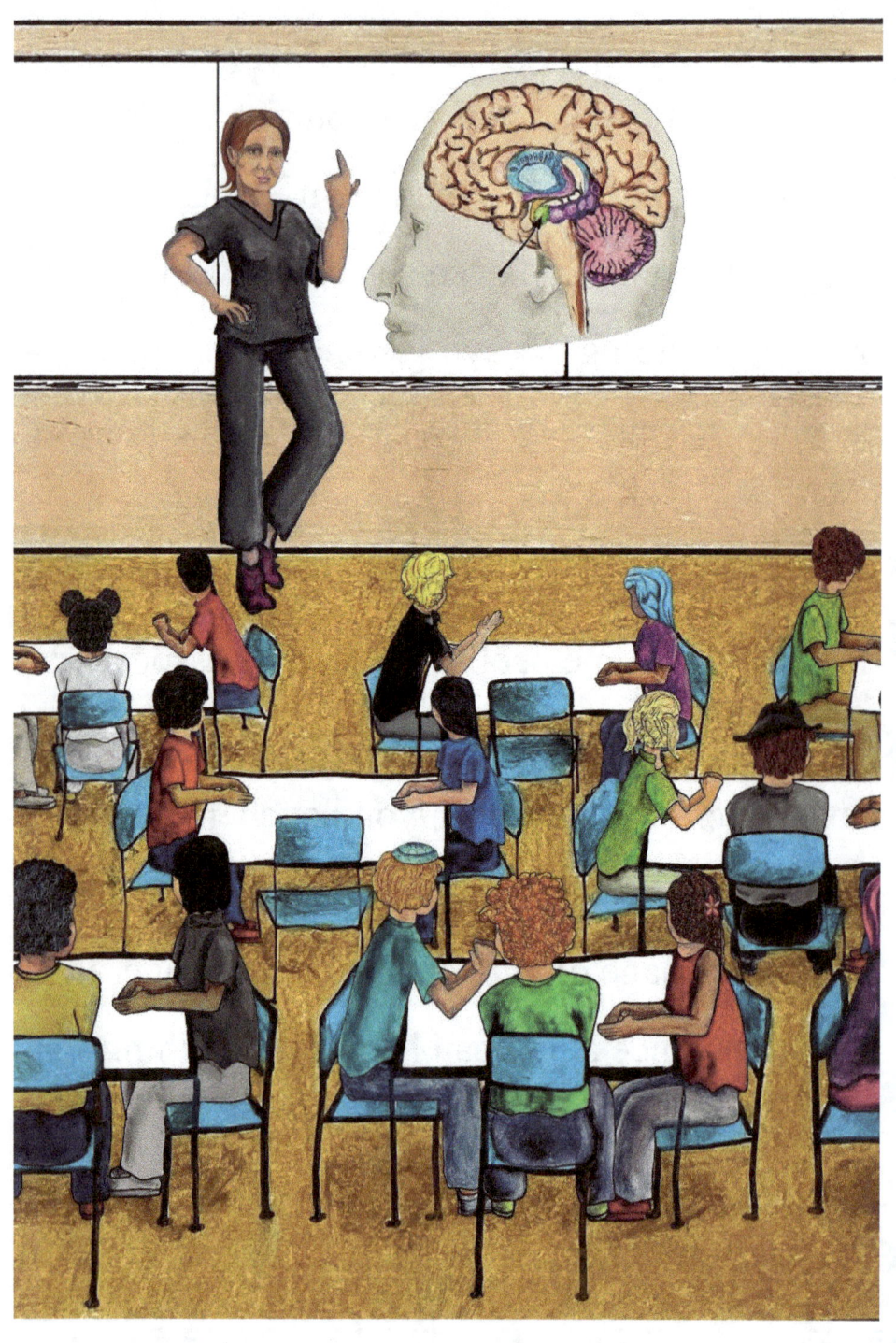

"The source of anger for humans is in the part of the brain called the amygdala, which the black line in the center is pointing to. It is the small green structure towards the bottom of the brain. When a person gets angry, they may have an increased heart rate. Their blood pressure may go up. The levels of certain hormones in the blood may increase, such as adrenaline from the adrenal glands. Anger can help motivate us to defend ourselves from danger. It can also alert us to something that has happened that appears to be unfair or unkind. We should not completely dismiss the emotion of anger since it was created for a reason. Learning to manage it can be difficult for some, especially if the person has a mood disorder. It's ok to ask for help from others, such as therapists, if you feel your anger is unmanageable."

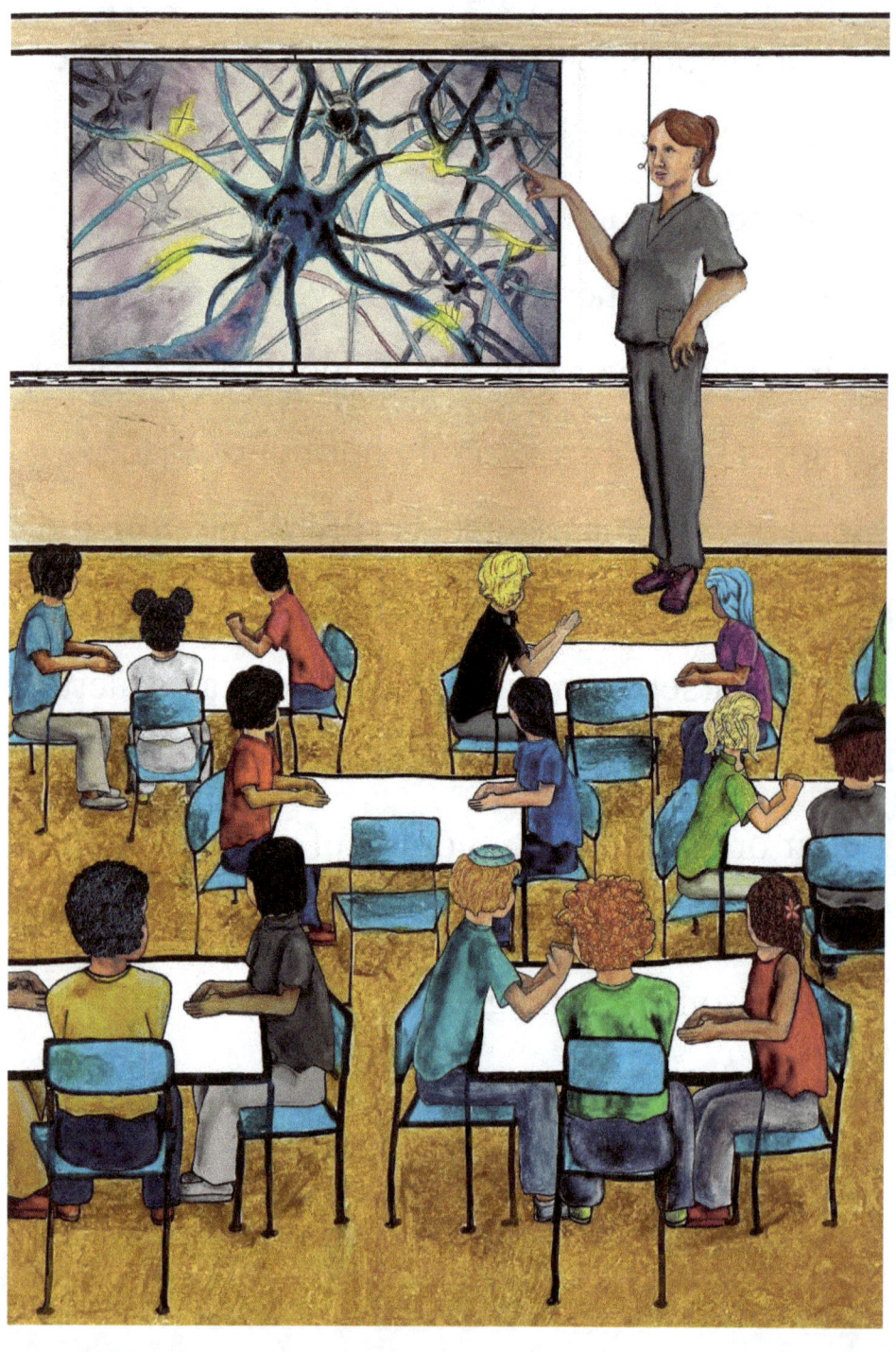

"Something that can help you manage your anger is knowing that the emotion is based on communications between different neurons in the brain. It is a biological process that could be affected by medications. Knowing that anger is the product of transmissions between neurons helps a person realize that the emotion is not a magical thing. Anger does not come from nowhere. Its existence is rooted in functions of the brain."

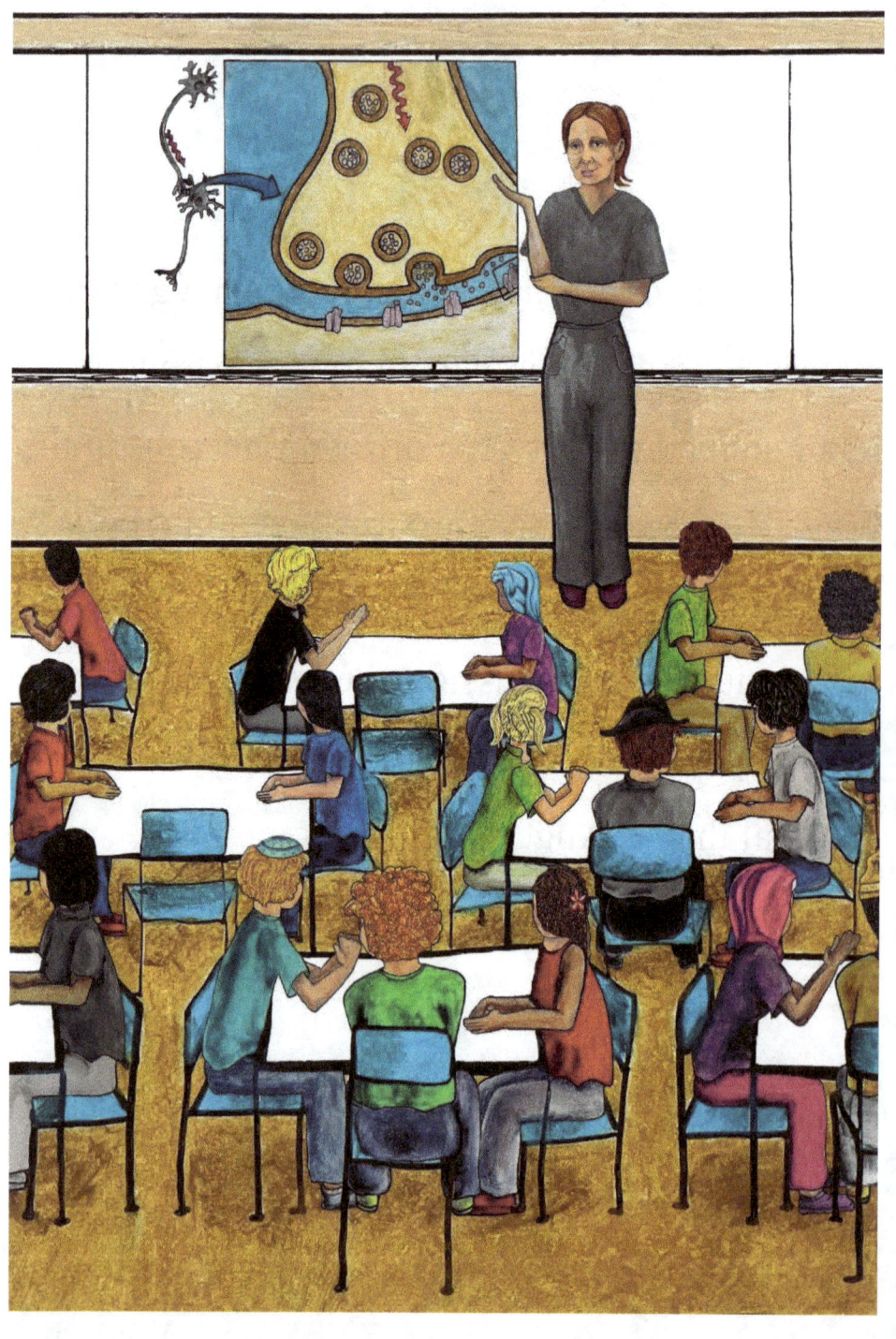

"Here's a close-up of the end of one neuron transmitting some neurotransmitters to another neuron. Medications can help adjust the levels of neurotransmitters which can affect the experience of anger. Some people with mood disorders require medicine to help live a normal life where anger is kept in check. Just like a person with diabetes will need some medication to live a physically healthy life, a person with a mood disorder may need medicine to live a mentally well life so that they can more easily manage their anger."

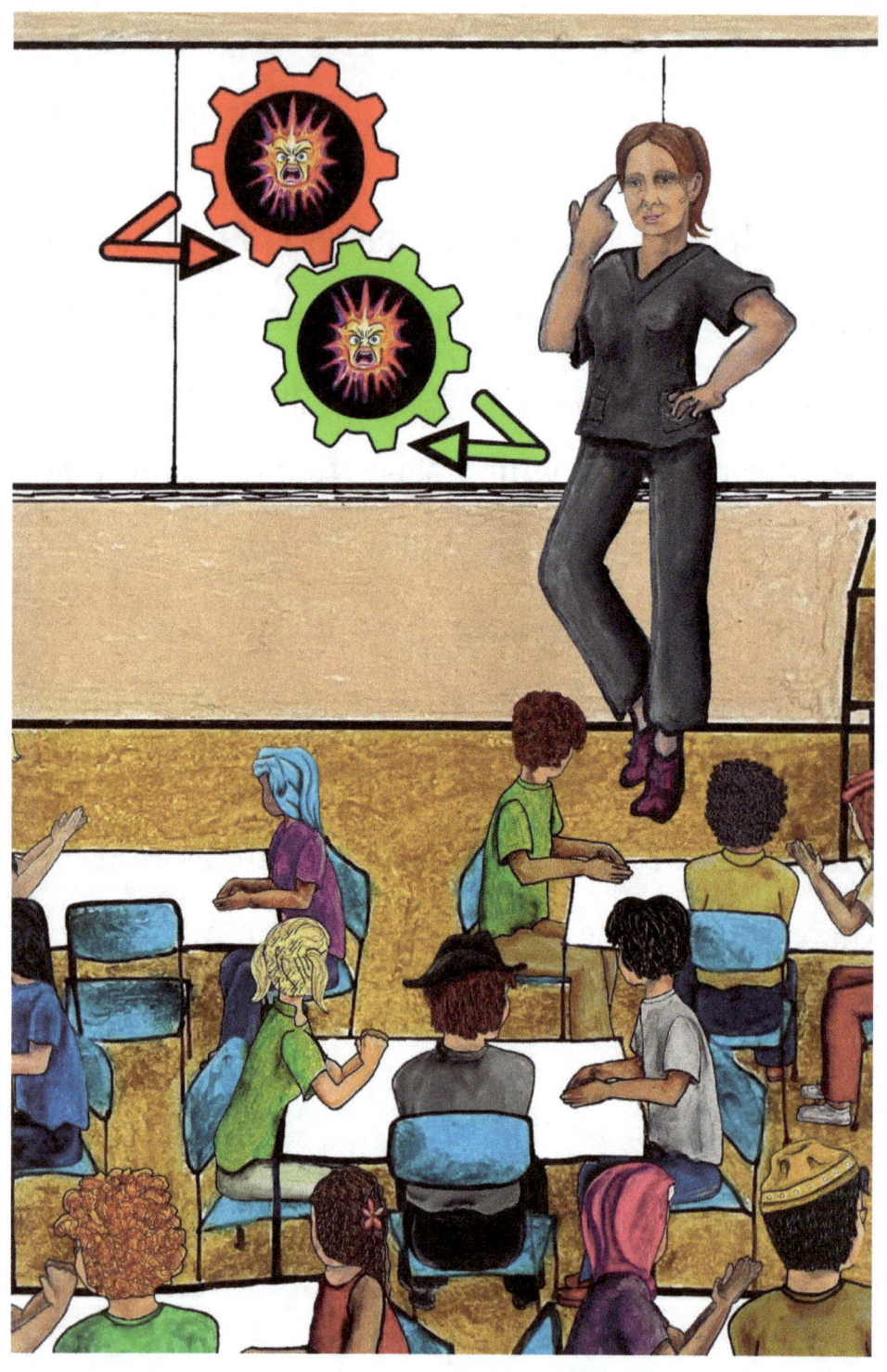

"Since anger is part of our survival mechanism when our life is threatened, we must face it and learn what triggers it. We must learn to use it in productive ways. We also must learn to manage it, since lashing out at everyone or everything that makes us angry is not acceptable to most social norms and cultures. Anger can destroy property. Anger can destroy relationships. Anger can lead to behaviors that can injure us. Anger can also lead to productivity to help others when they may be in trouble. Do not suppress your anger completely since it can be used to help many people."

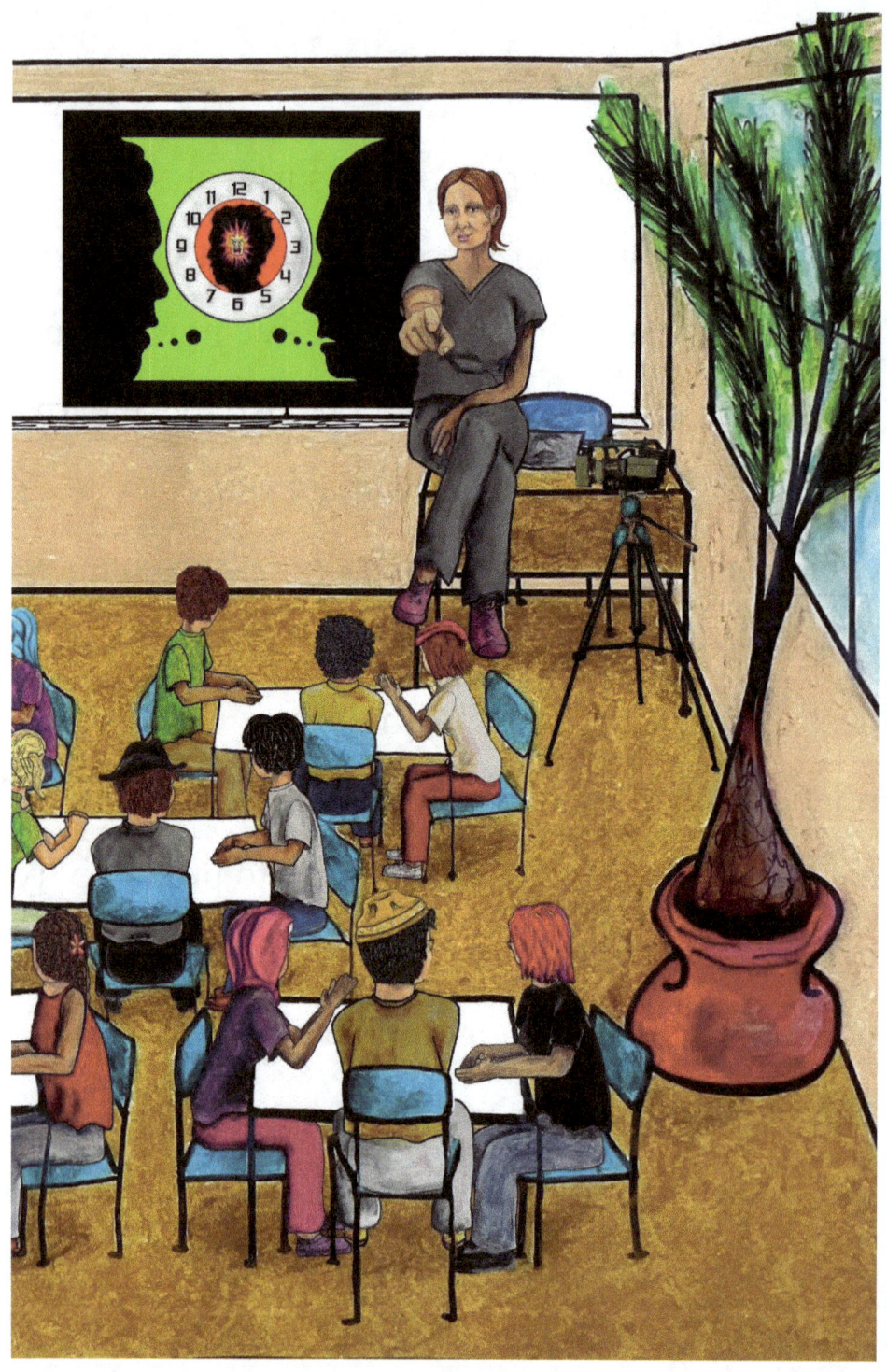

"Anger can be triggered by many different people, things, situations, memories, potential future events, and other things. Now, let's talk about some things that have made you angry. Share with those around you now, and we'll let you share with the class as you feel comfortable."

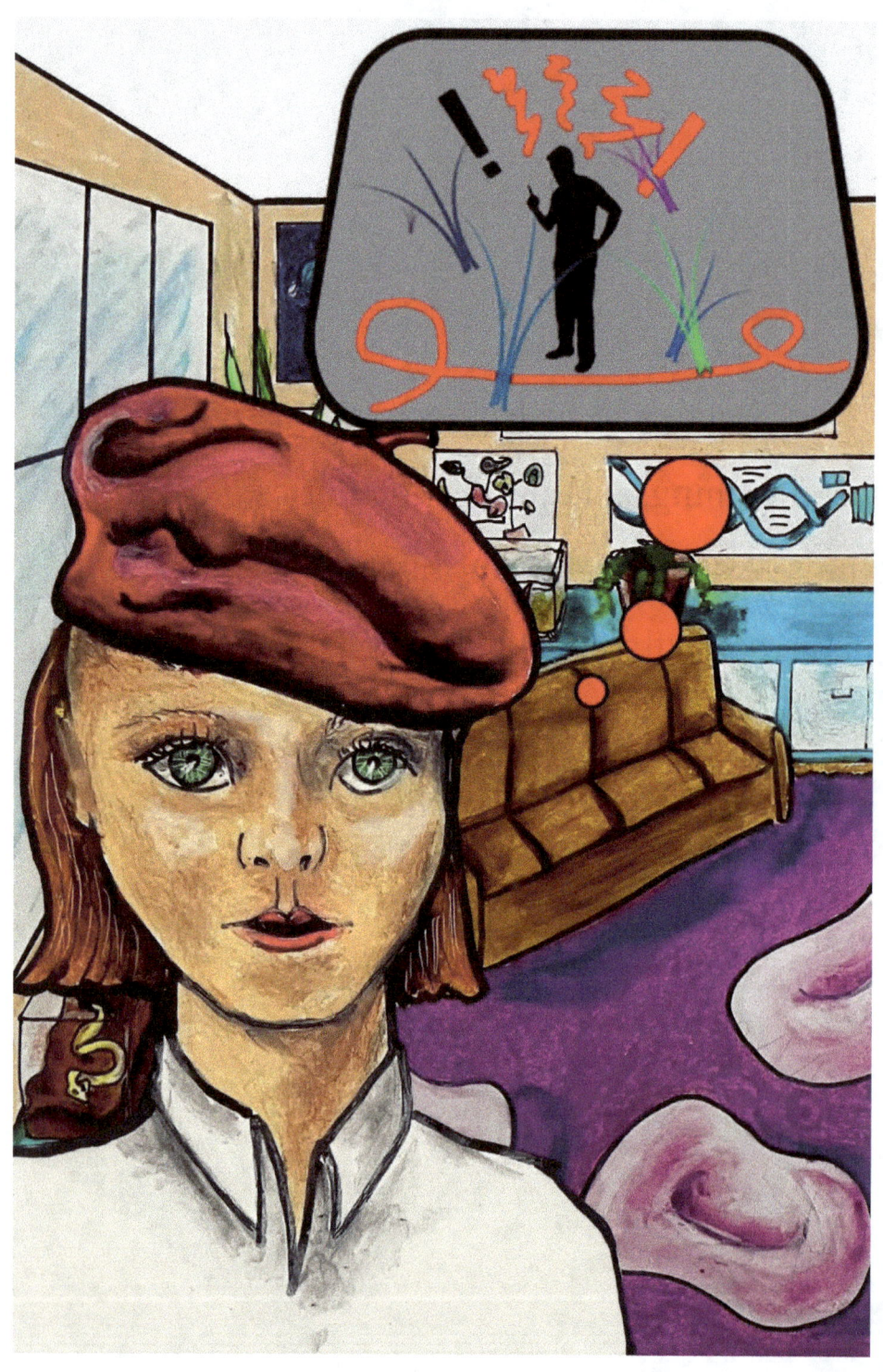

Marie raises her hand, and Nurse Dorothea calls on her to speak. "I have gotten frustrated with the progress of my garden. It seems to grow so slow and needs a lot of work. I wish the progress and growth would be quicker, but there's not much I can do."

"Progress can be slow with many things, including cultural progress, so that we all live in nurturing environments and that we are transformed into our best selves. Understanding the time it takes for things to develop and managing expectations can help reduce frustration," says Nurse Dorothea.

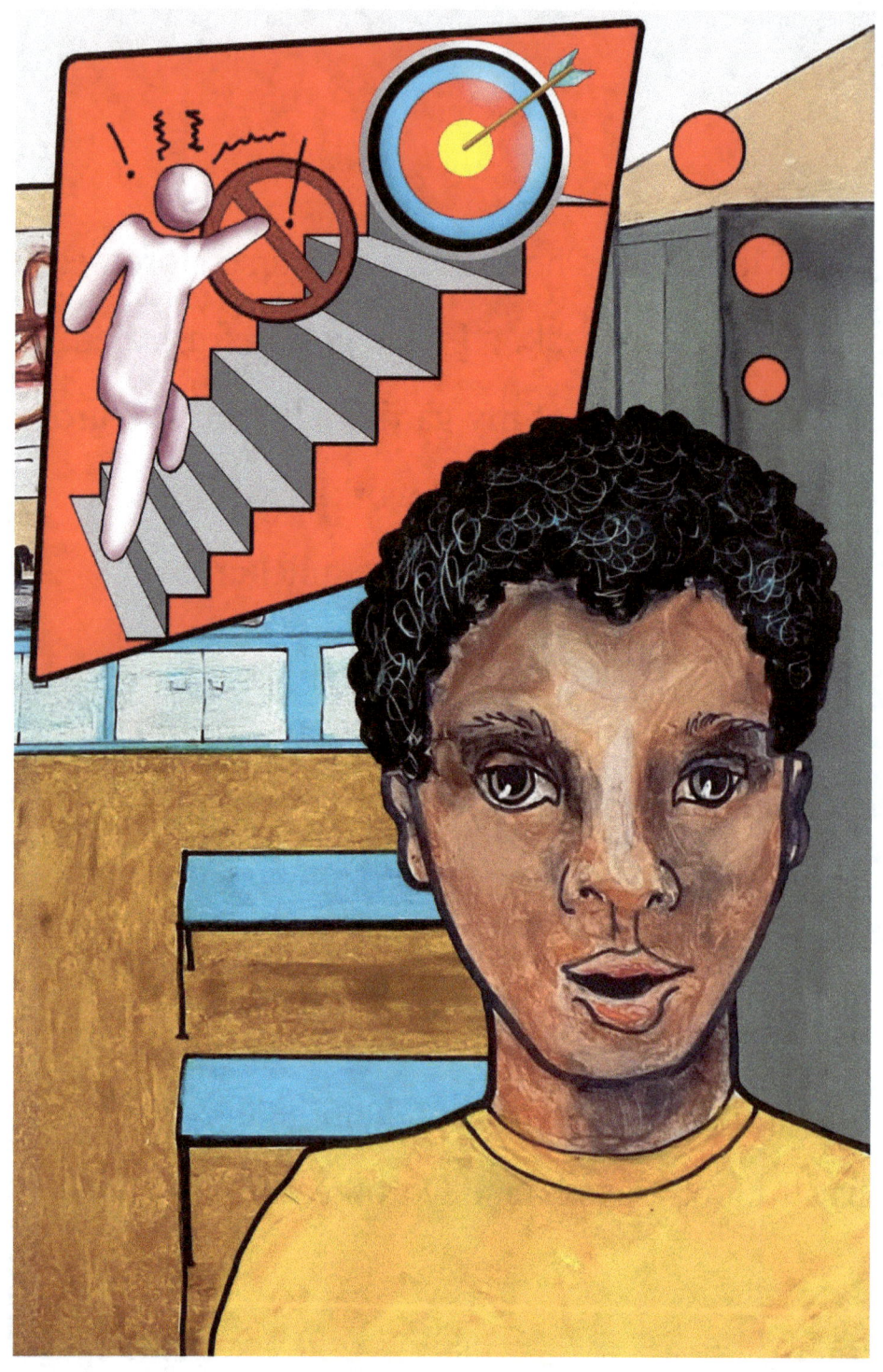

Ekon raises his hand, and Nurse Dorothea calls on him to speak. "When I set goals and things get in the way of me completing them, I get really frustrated. I want to succeed at whatever I start, and when I feel I can't accomplish and make achievements, then I get angry."

"Thanks for sharing. Your experience is normal. It may seem unfair to have obstacles in your way that seem to prevent you from accomplishing your goals. Understanding the complexity of our world can help manage anger since we can see things from a systems perspective and realize that some things are not what they appear to be. Not all obstacles are true obstacles since some things can help you develop your character," says Nurse Dorothea.

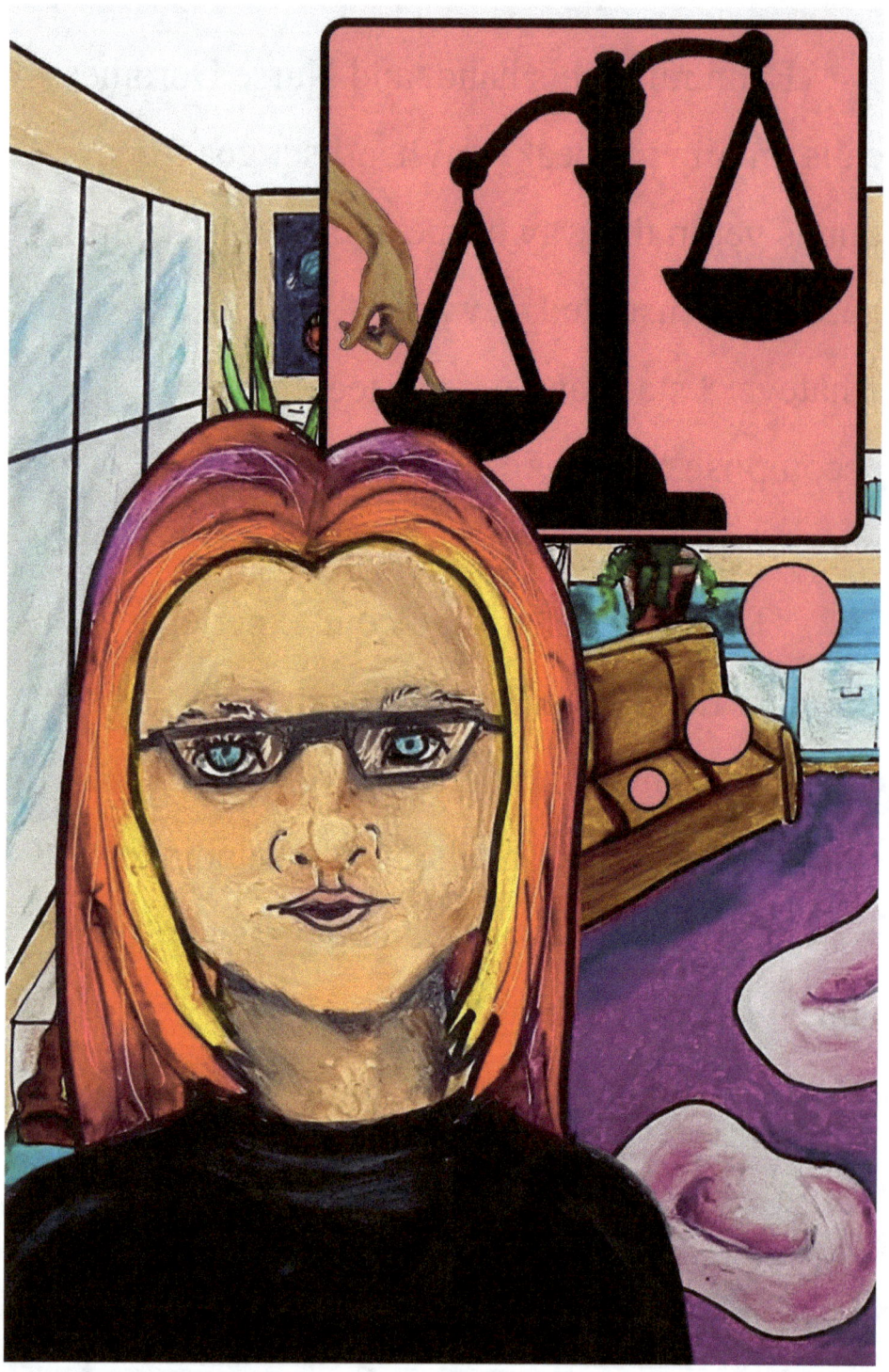

Juniper raises her hand, and Nurse Dorothea calls on her to speak. "When I see injustice, I get angry. When I watch short video clips of someone getting bullied or watch a movie and some injustice and violation of rights is happening, I get angry at the people I'm watching. I've even felt some hate toward some people in these videos."

"Seeing injustice is a trigger for anger for some people. I think we get angry because we don't want that unjust thing to happen to ourselves or to someone that we love. Fighting injustice in healthy and safe ways helps remove injustice from our culture," says Nurse Dorothea.

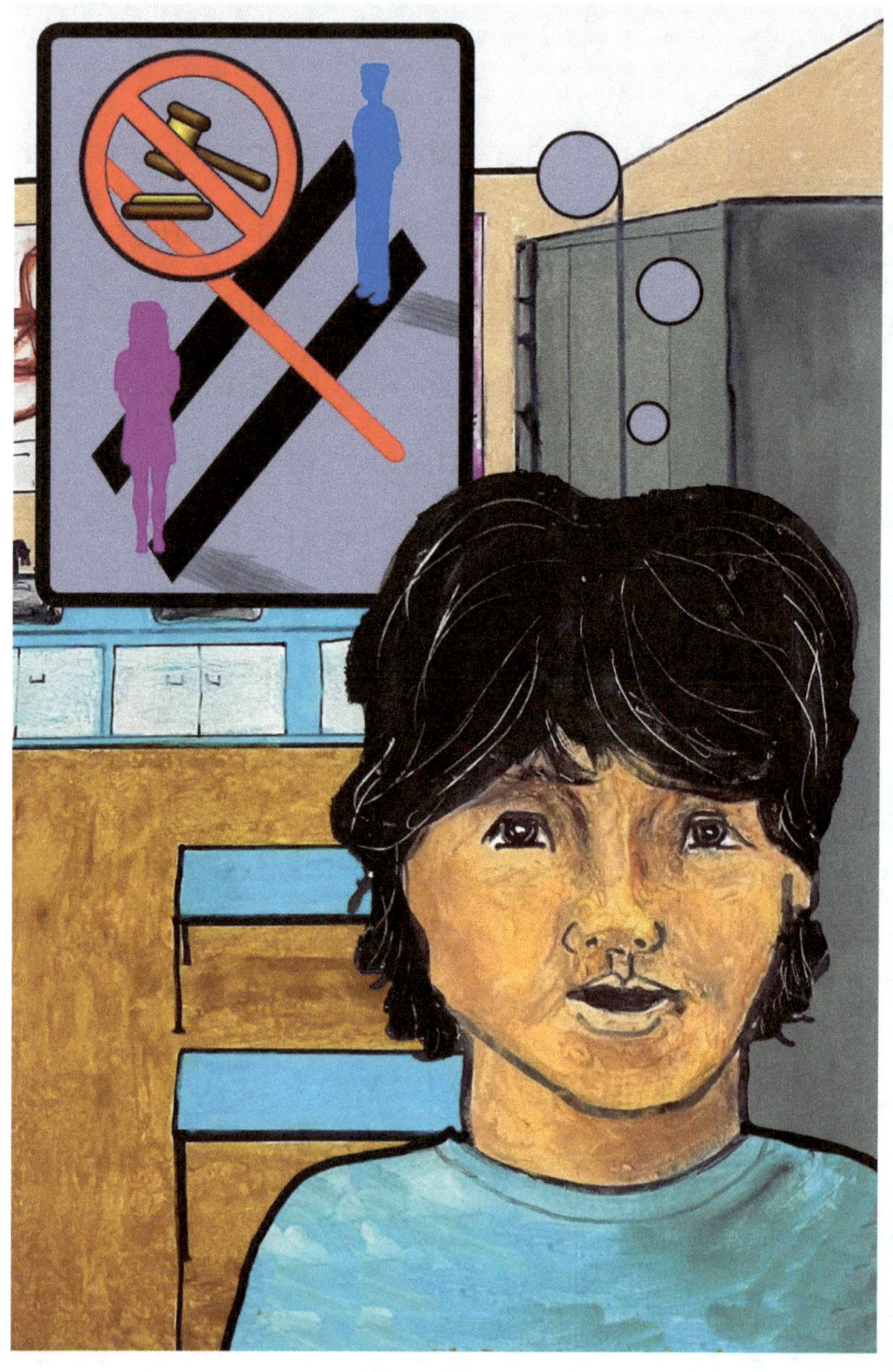

Ji Ho raises his hand, and Nurse Dorothea calls on him to speak. "I've seen unfair treatment in the past by a teacher where the teacher would yell at some people who were talking, but calmly and politely tell others to be quiet when they were talking. It seemed unfair that everyone wasn't treated the same. It made me upset, and I felt some anger, but I didn't know what to do."

"Even children seem to recognize when unfair treatment is occurring. It seems to be part of our DNA to recognize fairness in life, so we should all strive to display fair treatment to be good role models," says Nurse Dorothea.

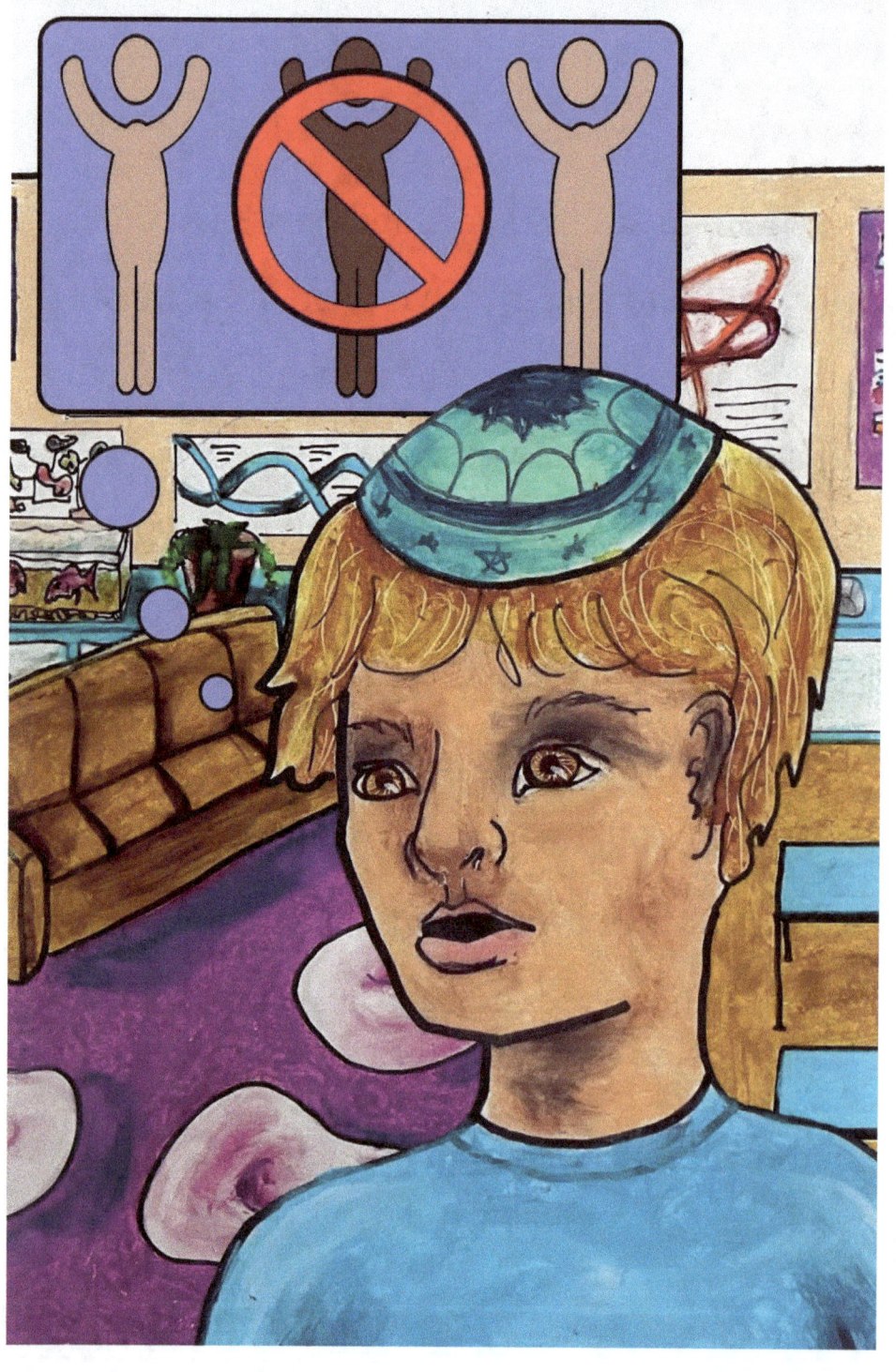

Levi raises his hand, and Nurse Dorothea calls on him to speak. "I get angry when I see discrimination based on human variations. I don't want people to be discriminated if they are disabled or based on the color of their skin. We are created by God and the Universe to be who we are, and we should not discriminate about something the person has no control over."

"There are laws in some countries to ban discrimination based on certain categories like race, religion, disability, and national origin. Again, cultural progress can be slow sometimes, but let's all do our part to be good role models and help our society be the best it can be," says Nurse Dorothea.

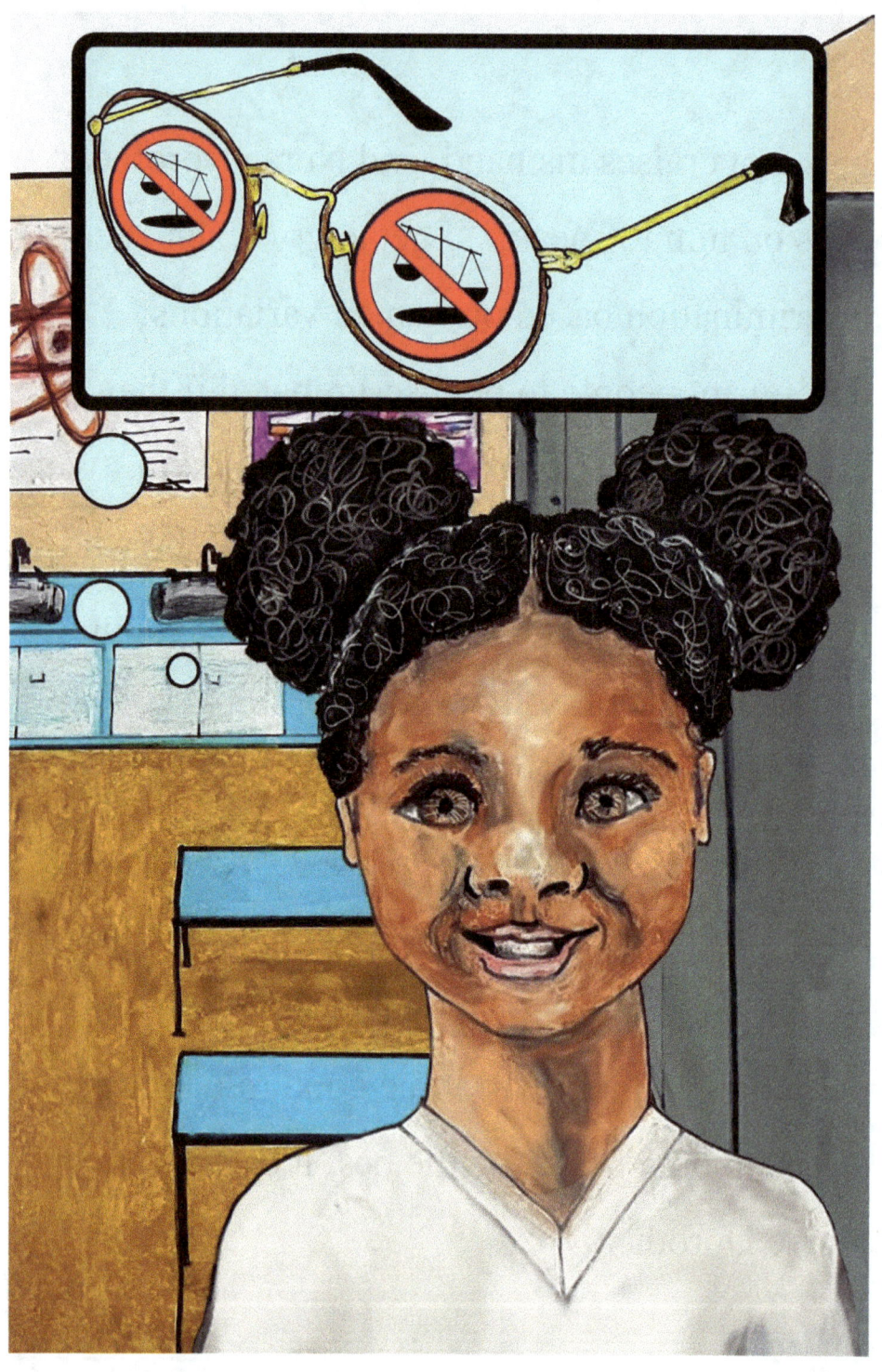

Amisha raises her hand, and Nurse Dorothea calls on her to speak. "Once I got angry about an injustice I perceived. I thought it was true and really happened. I talked to my mom about it, and we realized it was something I perceived, but was not true. I realized then that when I get angry about something, it is a good idea to talk to others about what I perceived, because maybe others didn't see it the same way. Understanding the injustice was only something I perceived, and that it was not real helped me release my anger and get back to peace."

"That was great. You gained the insight that we need to talk to others sometimes about our anger to see if we were angry over an observable fact. Triggers of anger can be real and can also be in one's perception only," says Nurse Dorothea.

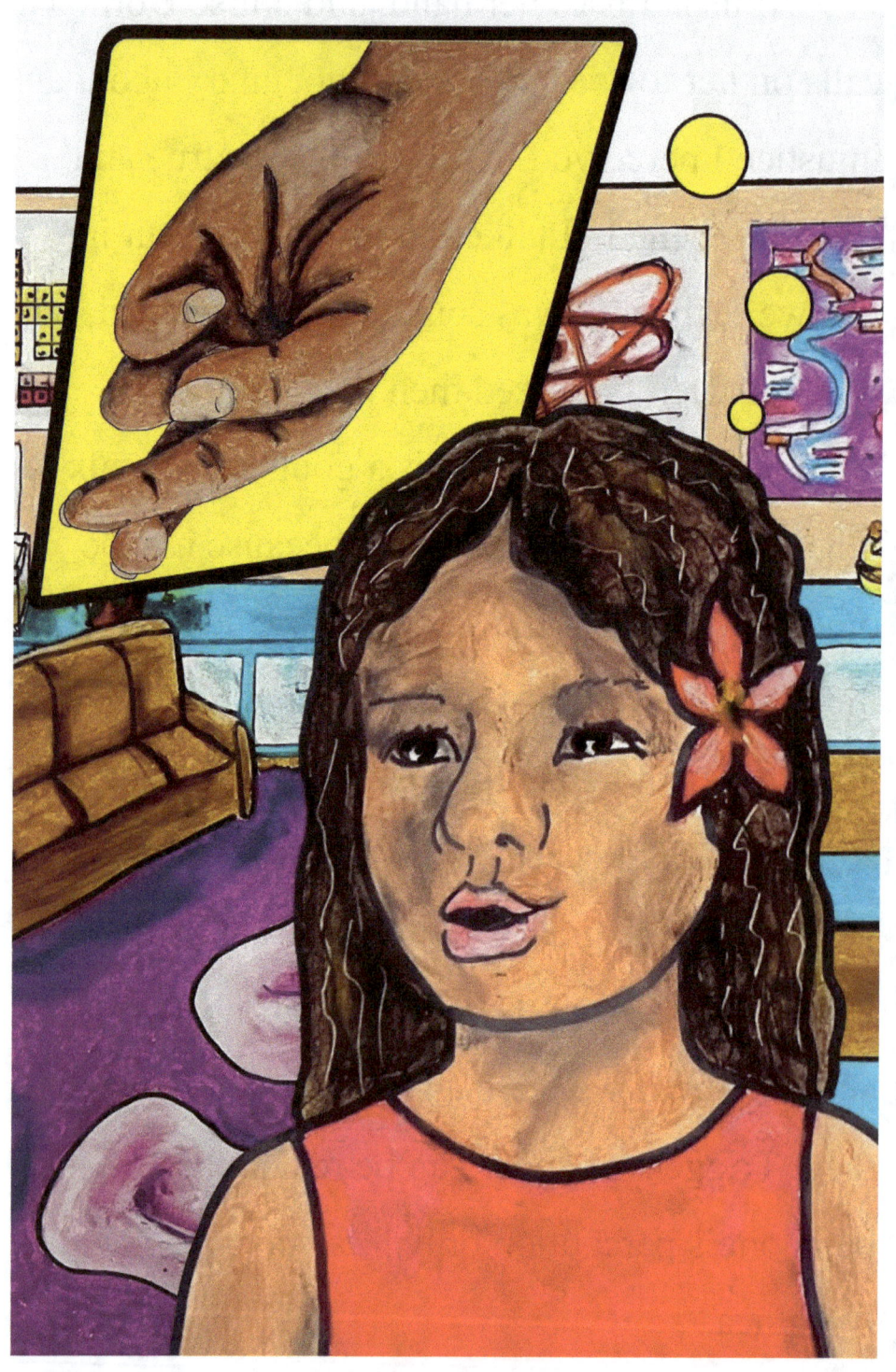

Kalani raises her hand, and Nurse Dorothea calls on her to speak. "I was lied to by someone I considered a friend, and I got very angry."

"Being lied to can create a feeling of betrayal which can trigger anger. We need to try to develop open and welcoming relationships with others so that they don't feel the need to lie to us. Lying can harm others even though it is just words," says Nurse Dorothea.

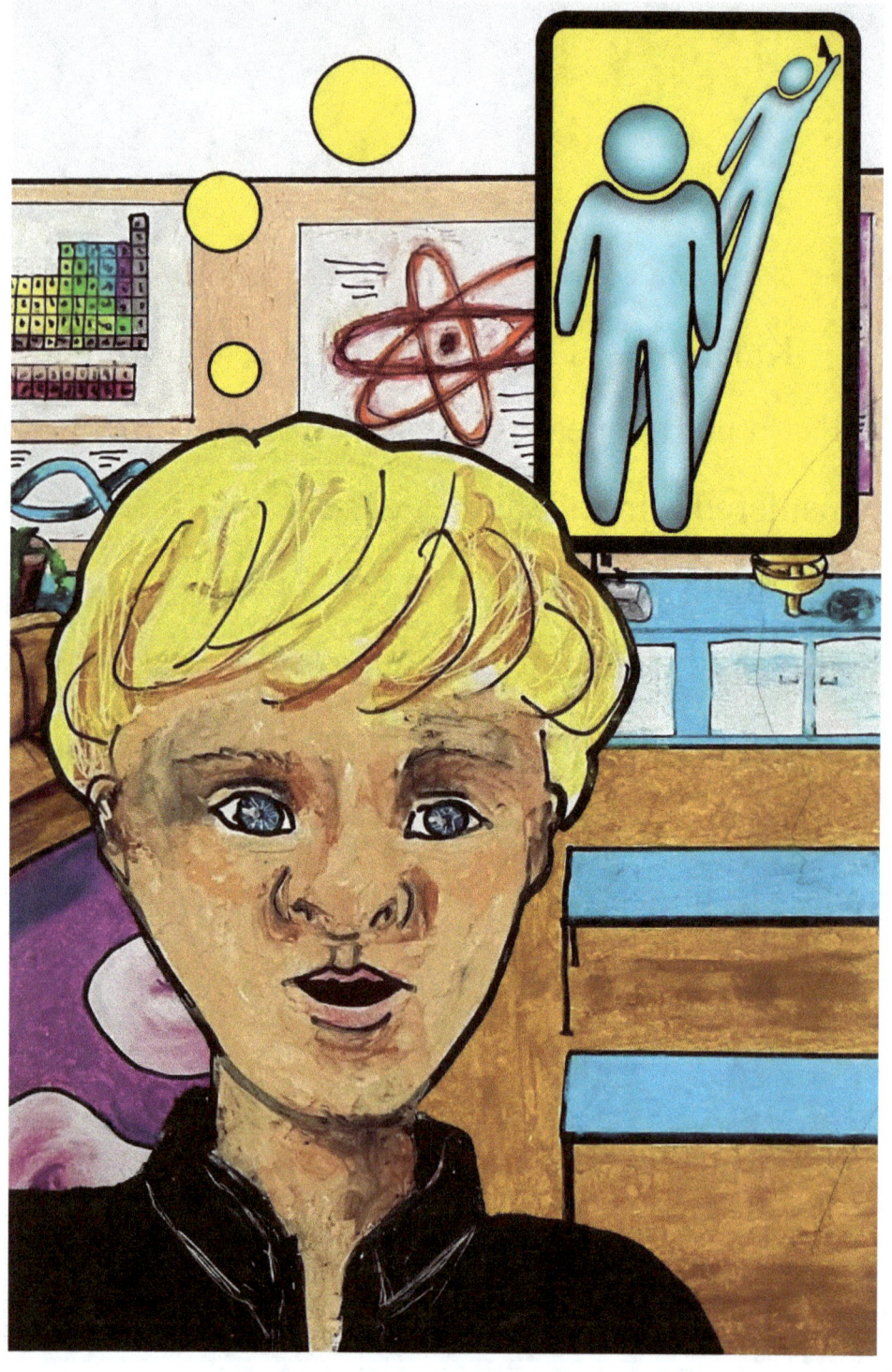

Dimitry raises his hand, and Nurse Dorothea calls on him to speak. "I was deceived once. I researched deception and discovered that it is the practice of making someone accept as true something false or invalid. It made me angry that I accepted what was false as true. It messed with my mind and disturbed me. I just want to learn and live in the truth."

"Being deceived can make us feel like a fool and trigger our anger. Let's all try not to deceive each other," says Nurse Dorothea.

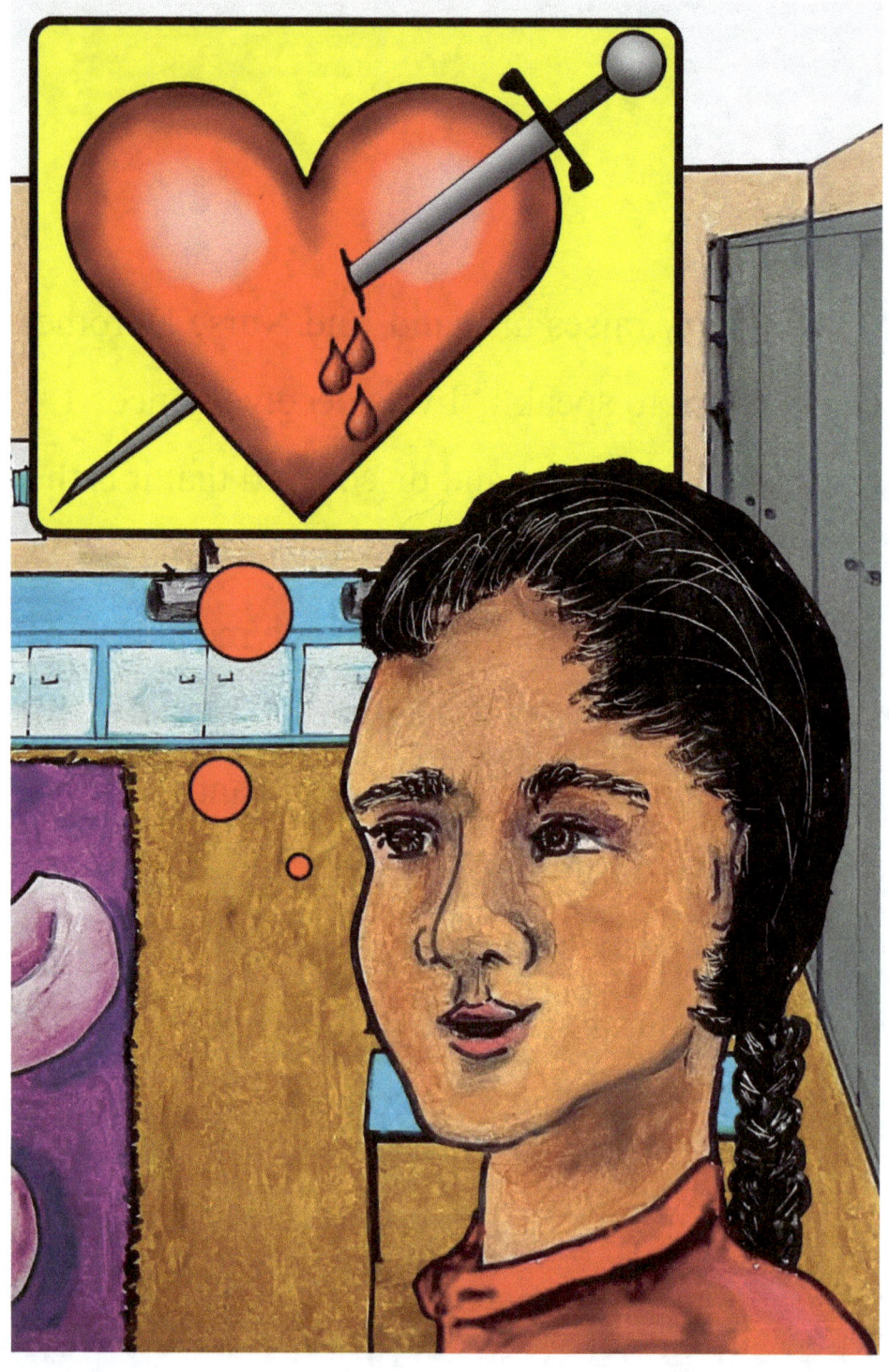

Pia raises her hand, and Nurse Dorothea calls on her to speak. "I had a friend betray me by stealing my ex-boyfriend from me. It made me cry a lot, and then I became very angry at both of them. It made me be more cautious about who I let get close to me."

"Betrayal can cause people to isolate themselves and stop communicating with other loved ones. I would say your old friend took you for granted and didn't appreciate your friendship. We need to learn not to take others for granted since it can affect many people," says Nurse Dorothea.

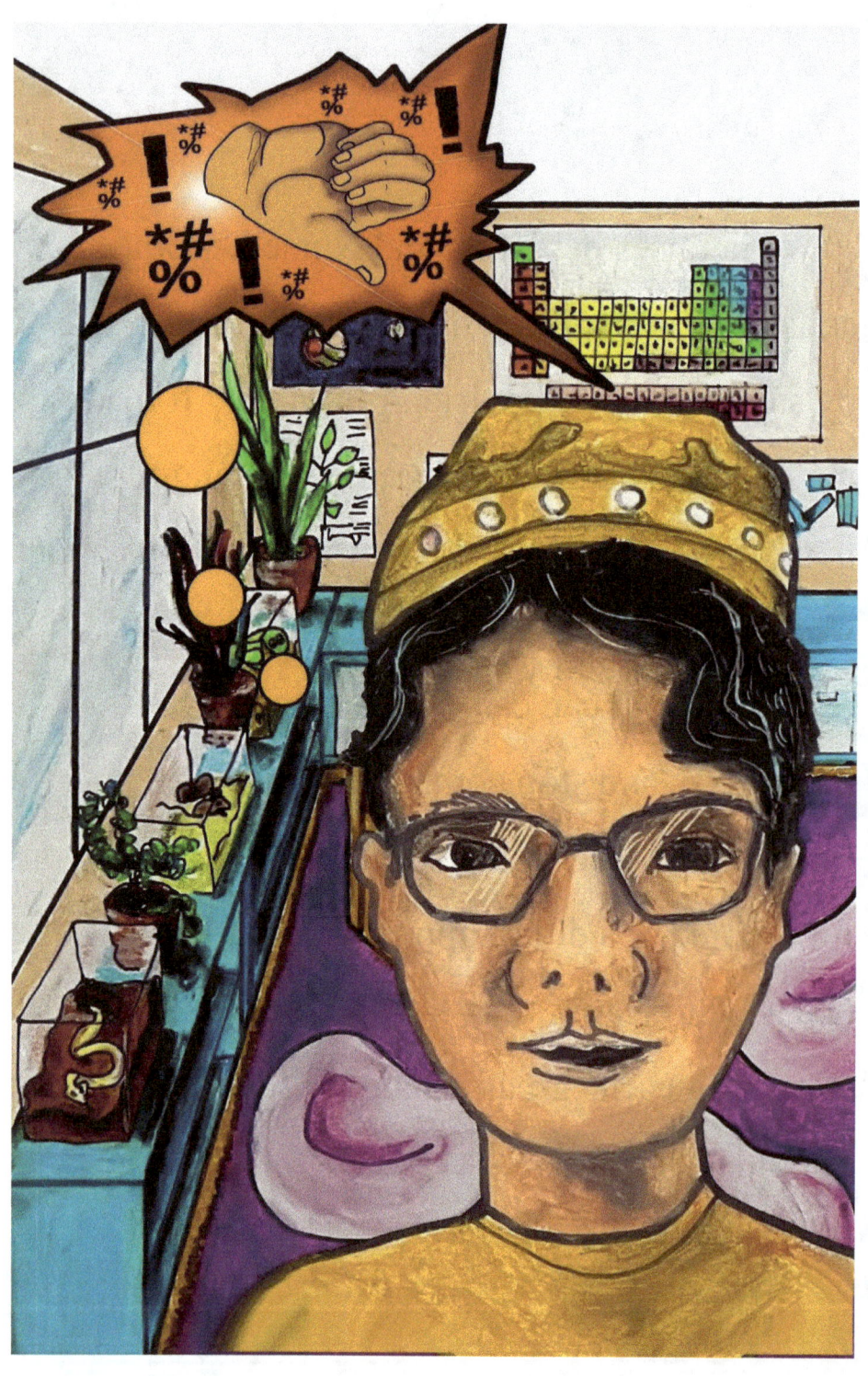

Azamat raises his hand, and Nurse Dorothea calls on him to speak. "I was shopping one day, and the workers were disrespecting me and choosing not to help me. I think it was because I was a teenager, and maybe they thought I wasn't going to buy anything. It made me frustrated, and I left. My mom later told me I should have talked to the supervisor to get help."

"Advocating for yourself with assertiveness is important when you feel disrespected. Say what you mean, mean what you say, and don't say it mean," says Nurse Dorothea.

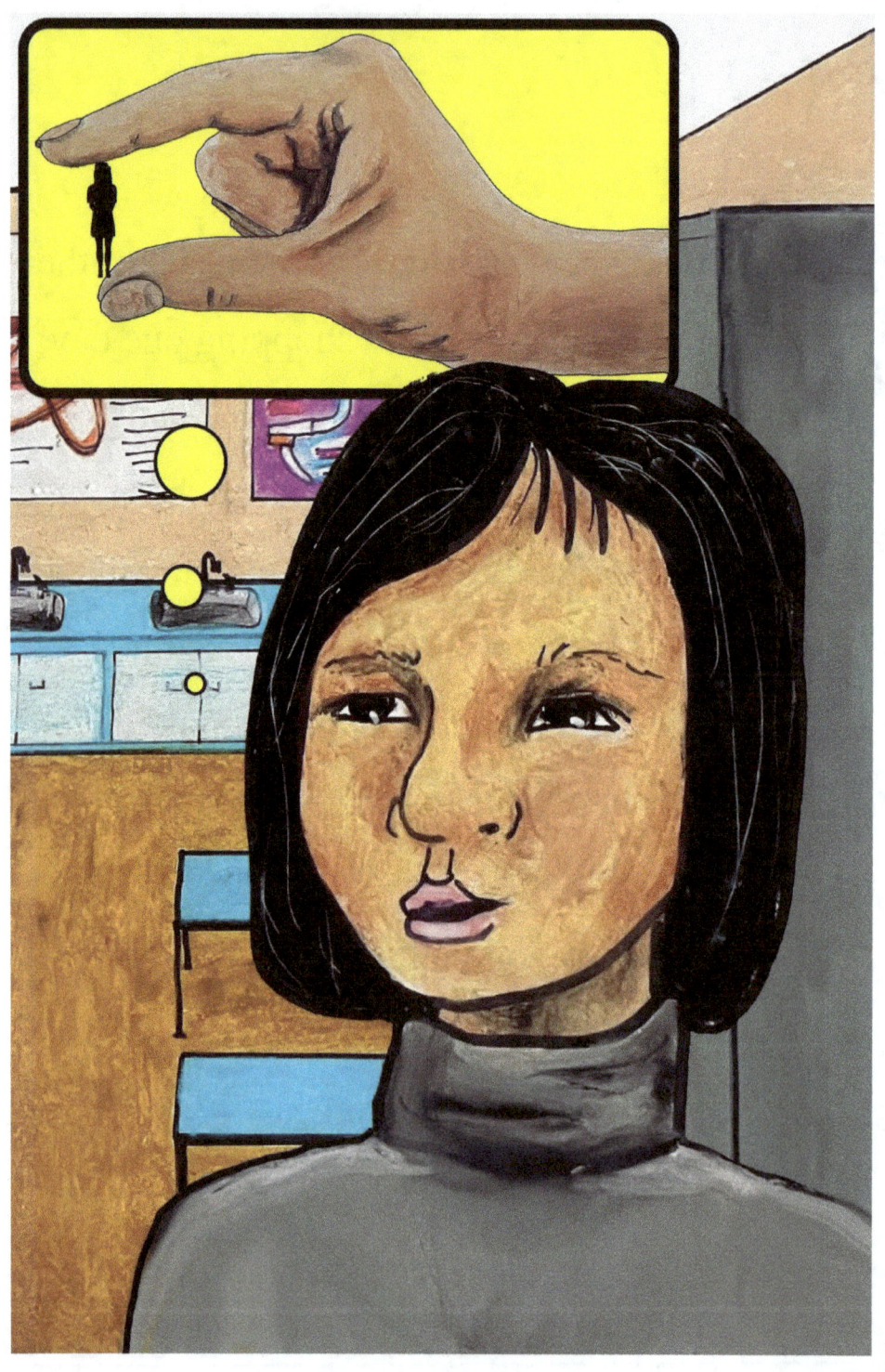

Lian raises her hand, and Nurse Dorothea calls on her to talk. "Someone once said things to make me feel little and unimportant. It felt hurtful and made me feel bad. Later, as I was thinking about it, I realized they were wrong to have said that, and it made me angry."

"For some reason, we have lived in a world where making others feel small and unimportant is normalized. Maybe one day, we will live in a world where we are all seen as important and key to our civilization's future. A human being's creation is a miracle, and an incredible amount of evolution was involved to get us to be the people we are today. Let us maintain hope of a future free of discrimination based on natural characteristics, and where we are all on a trajectory of ever-increasing potential," says Nurse Dorothea.

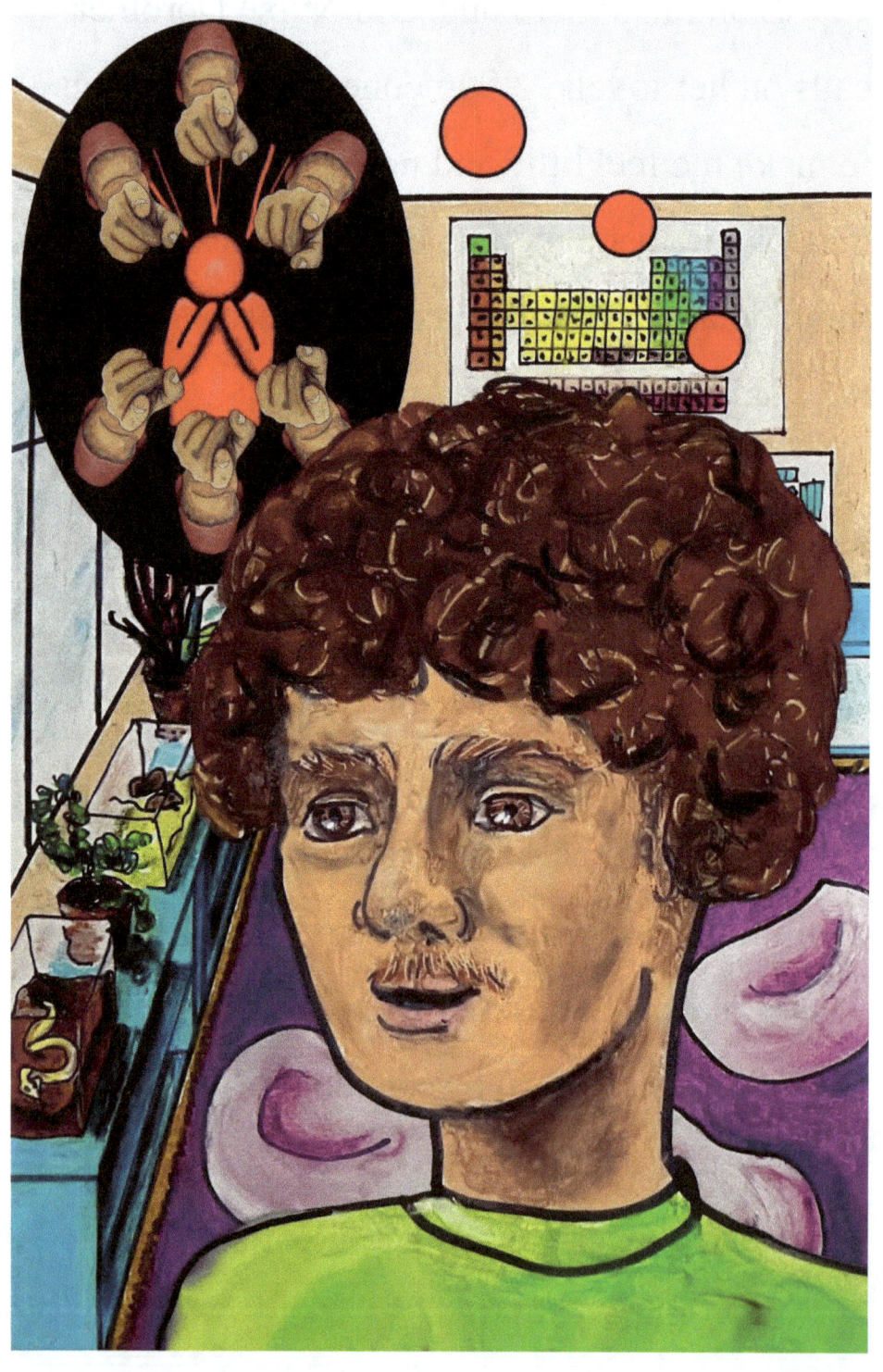

Gustavo raises his hand, and Nurse Dorothea calls on him to talk. "I did something embarrassing once and was then humiliated by many people who saw what I did. I felt horrible, and then later, I felt angry for being humiliated in front of so many people. I felt ashamed, and then I had thoughts of trying to humiliate those who said those mean things."

"Sometimes anger can cause us to seek revenge and do the same things back to those who did something mean to us. Let us seek the higher ground and improve our own nature as well as those around us. Let us live transformative lives," says Nurse Dorothea.

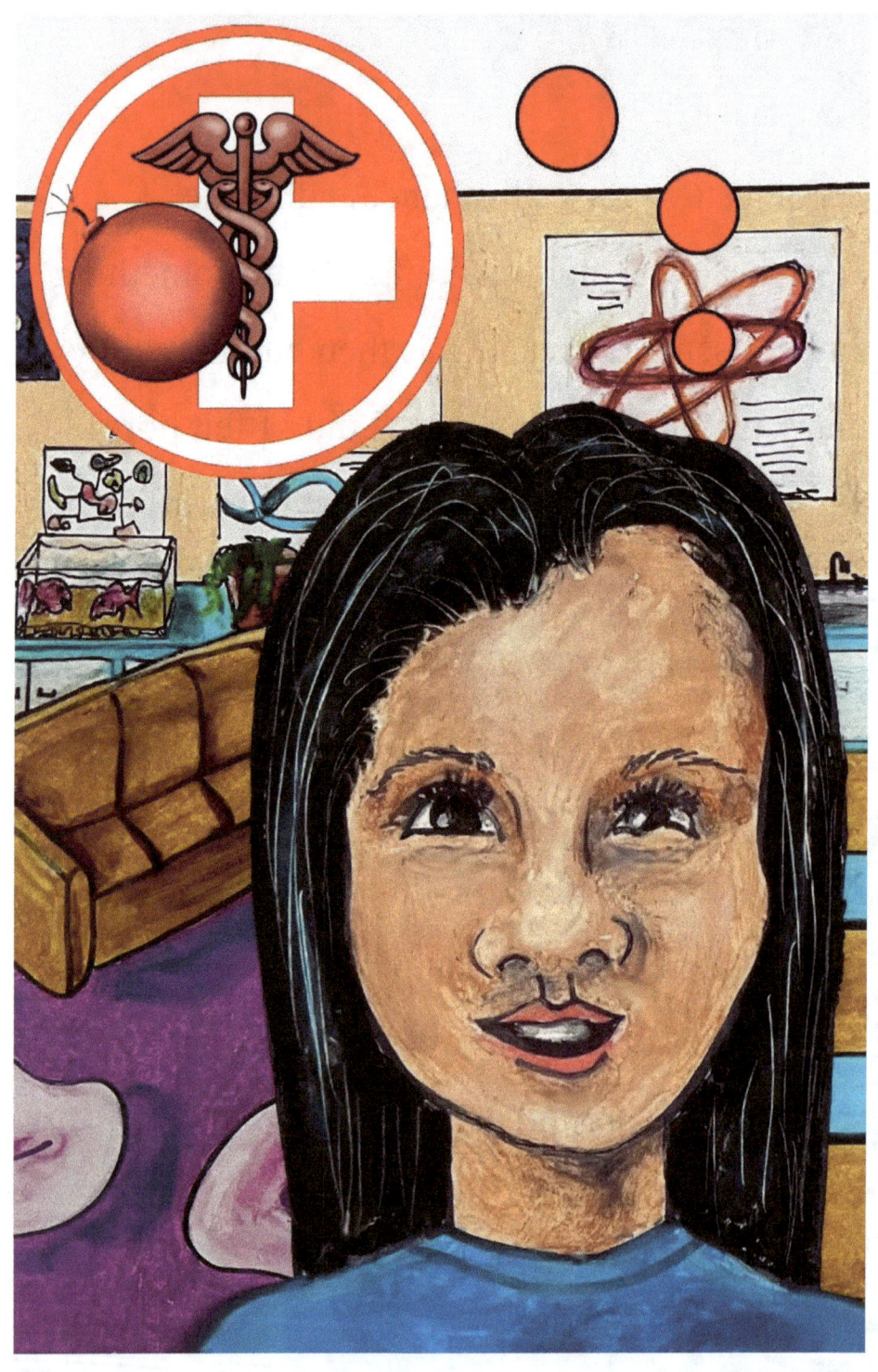

Diwa raises her hand, and Nurse Dorothea calls on her to talk. "Once, I was in a very bad situation and my physical safety was threatened. It is something I still have PTSD about. Someone was robbing the convenience store with a gun, and I felt my life was in danger, even though I was there just to buy a drink. I was very scared. As the weeks went by after the event, I became angry at the world for letting me be in that situation."

"Some people can get very angry immediately when their physical safety is in danger, so that is why anger is dangerous since many people can be harmed during a threatening event, even bystanders. When rage comes through a person, he or she must be very careful, since they may do things that might put their physical safety in more danger," says Nurse Dorothea.

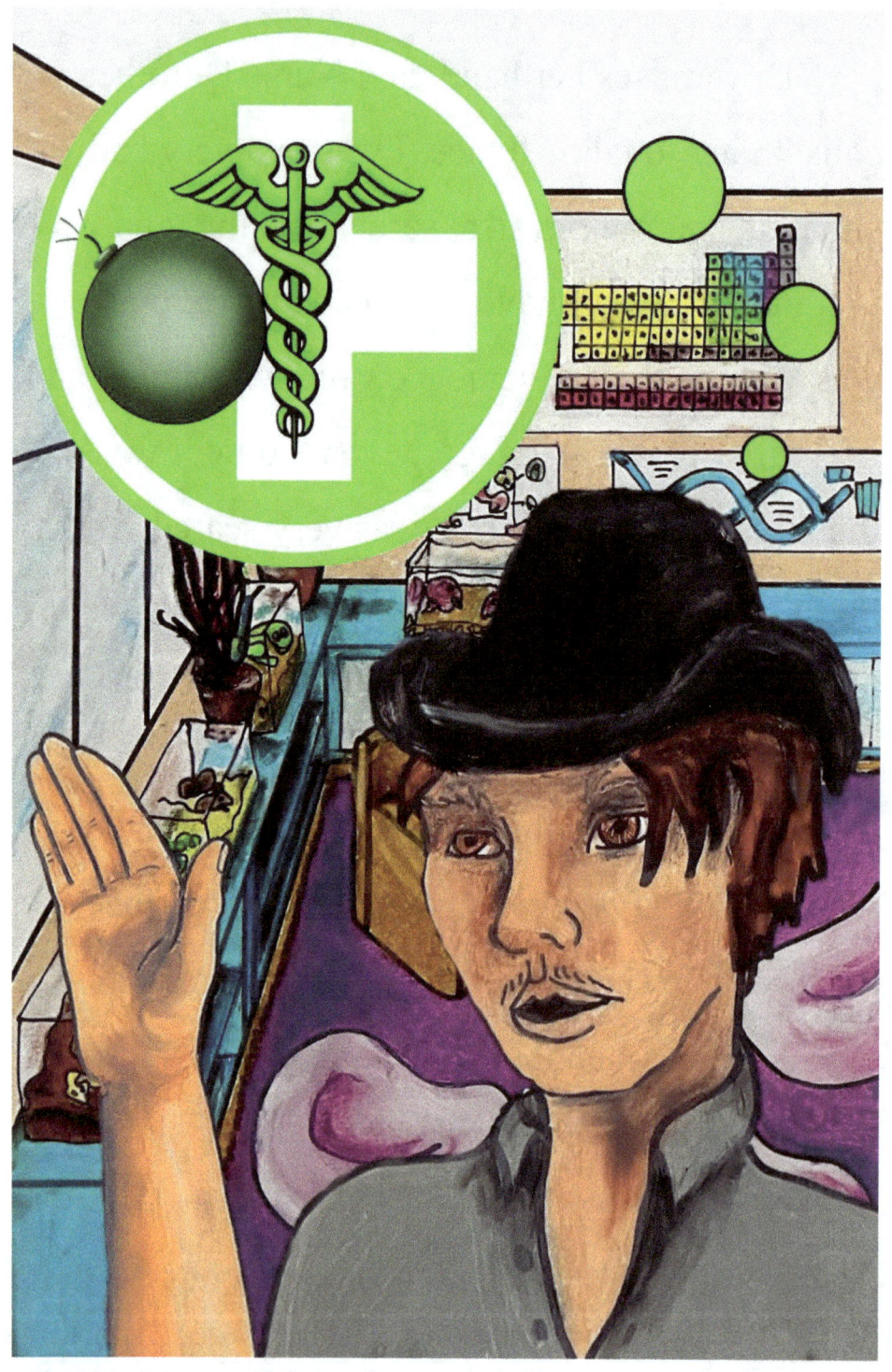

Wyatt raises his hand, and Nurse Dorothea calls on him to talk. "I get frustrated when I get yelled at by family members for no good reason because I feel my emotional safety is at risk."

"Good communication is a skill, and all humans need to develop it so that we can provide a safe place for all using effective and helpful words," says Nurse Dorothea.

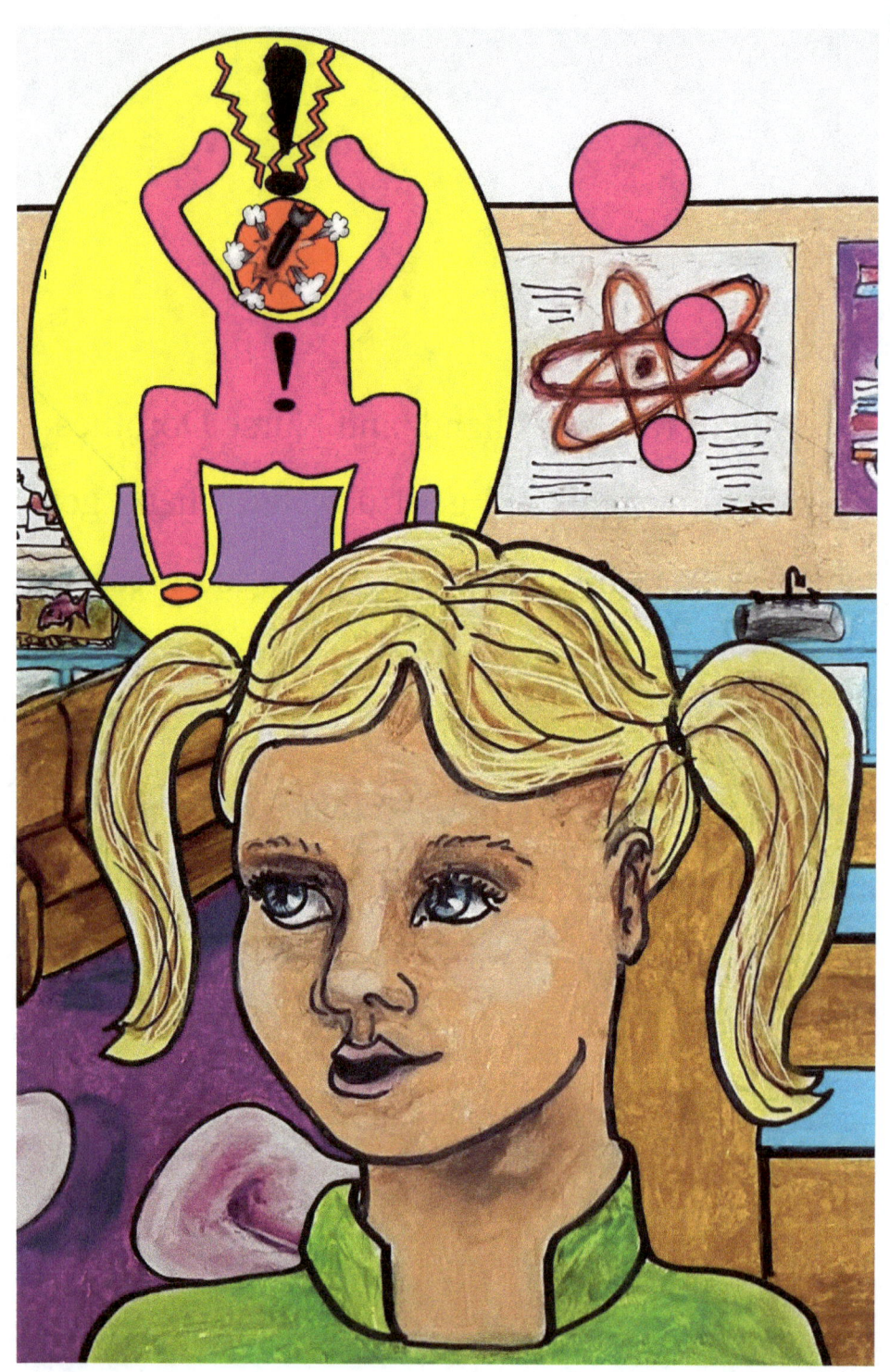

Frida raises her hand, and Nurse Dorothea calls on her to talk. "I have PTSD from something that happened to me a couple of years ago. I don't want to talk about what happened, but when certain kinds of people say certain things to me, it triggers all the emotions to come back. I'm angry because I worry I'll have to deal with PTSD for the rest of my life."

"Post traumatic stress disorder or PTSD is a real thing and can affect a person's life. Getting therapy can help and there is even a medication that can help with nightmares if you have those. Talk to your doctor about the right treatment for you," says Nurse Dorothea.

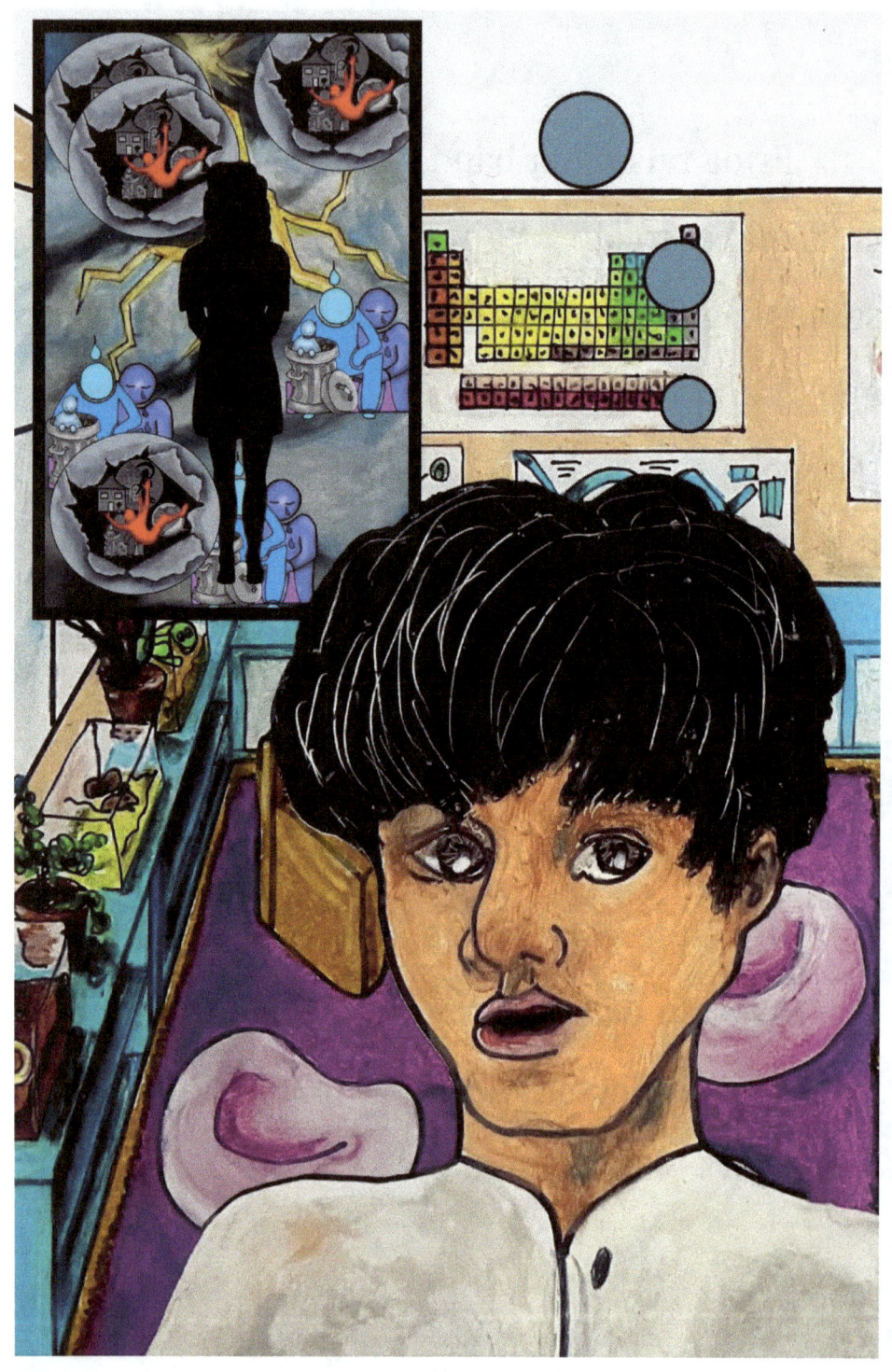

Antonio raises his hand, and Nurse Dorothea calls on him to talk. "After I get feelings of depression, the depression seems to turn into anger about the things I get depressed about."

"That's an example of how emotions are on a spectrum, and one can lead into another. Some people need mood medication, and a psychiatrist can help with that," says Nurse Dorothea.

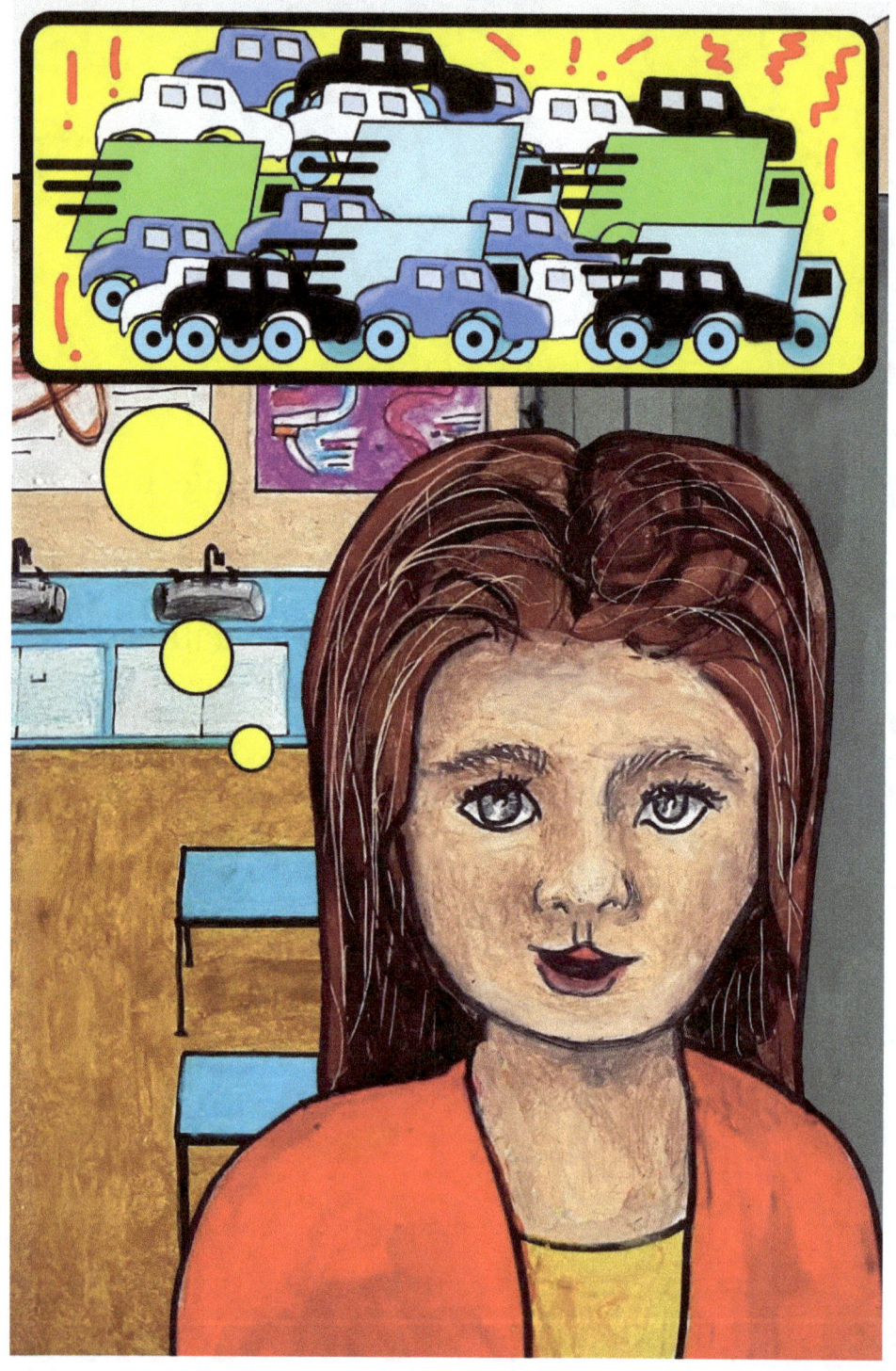

Awira raises her hand, and Nurse Dorothea calls on her to talk. "I really get frustrated when my family gets into a traffic jam while we are trying to get to places like school. It's so frustrating to just sit in the same place for a while until the cars start moving again."

"Everyday life can frustrate people sometimes, so that is why we need to recognize our emotions. We need to learn to manage them, so that they don't manage us," says Nurse Dorothea.

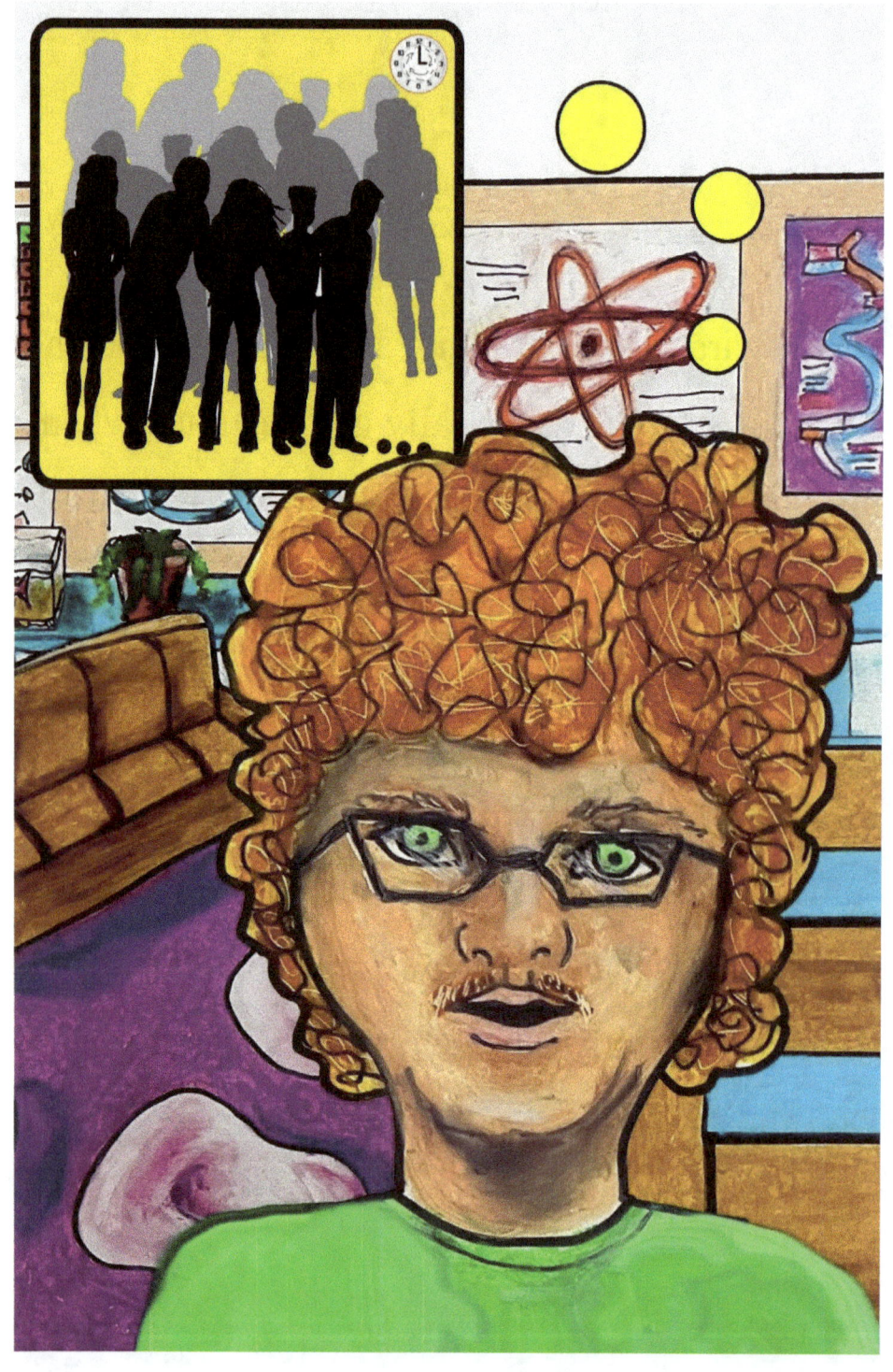

Connor raises his hand, and Nurse Dorothea calls on him to talk. "I get frustrated about another everyday thing such as waiting in lines at stores. I feel my time is being wasted."

"Again, everyday situations can lead to frustration, which is why we need to develop healthy coping skills. While we wait in lines, we could use our technology to listen to music we love, read a book on our phone, or other things, including calling a friend we haven't talked to in a while. Coping skills need to be developed for frustration, anger, and rage," says Nurse Dorothea.

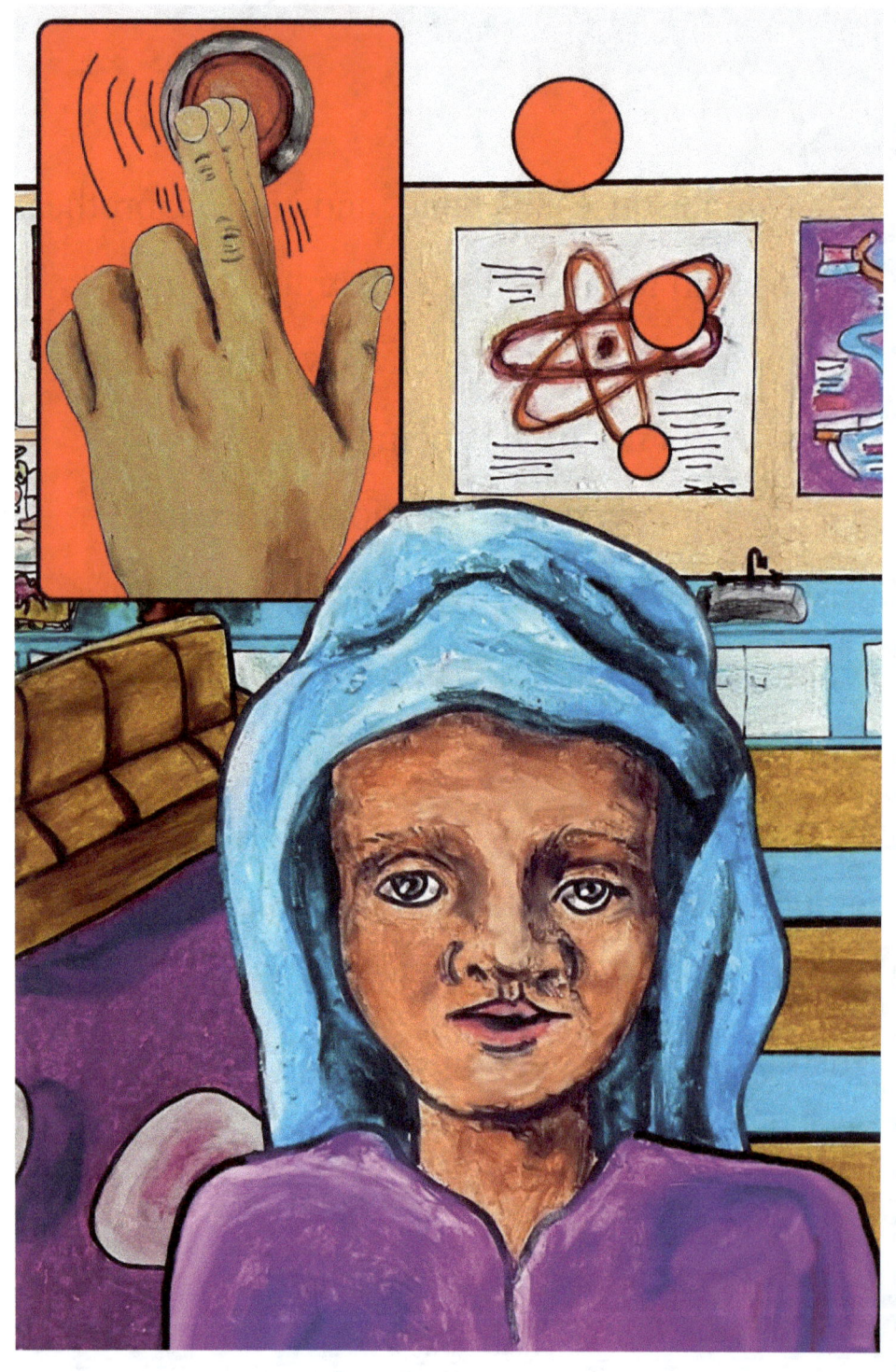

Yuliana raises her hand, and Nurse Dorothea calls on her to talk. "Repetitive things annoy me such as someone ringing the doorbell over and over."

"Things that repeat can be frustrating, and we need to understand our triggers," says Nurse Dorothea.

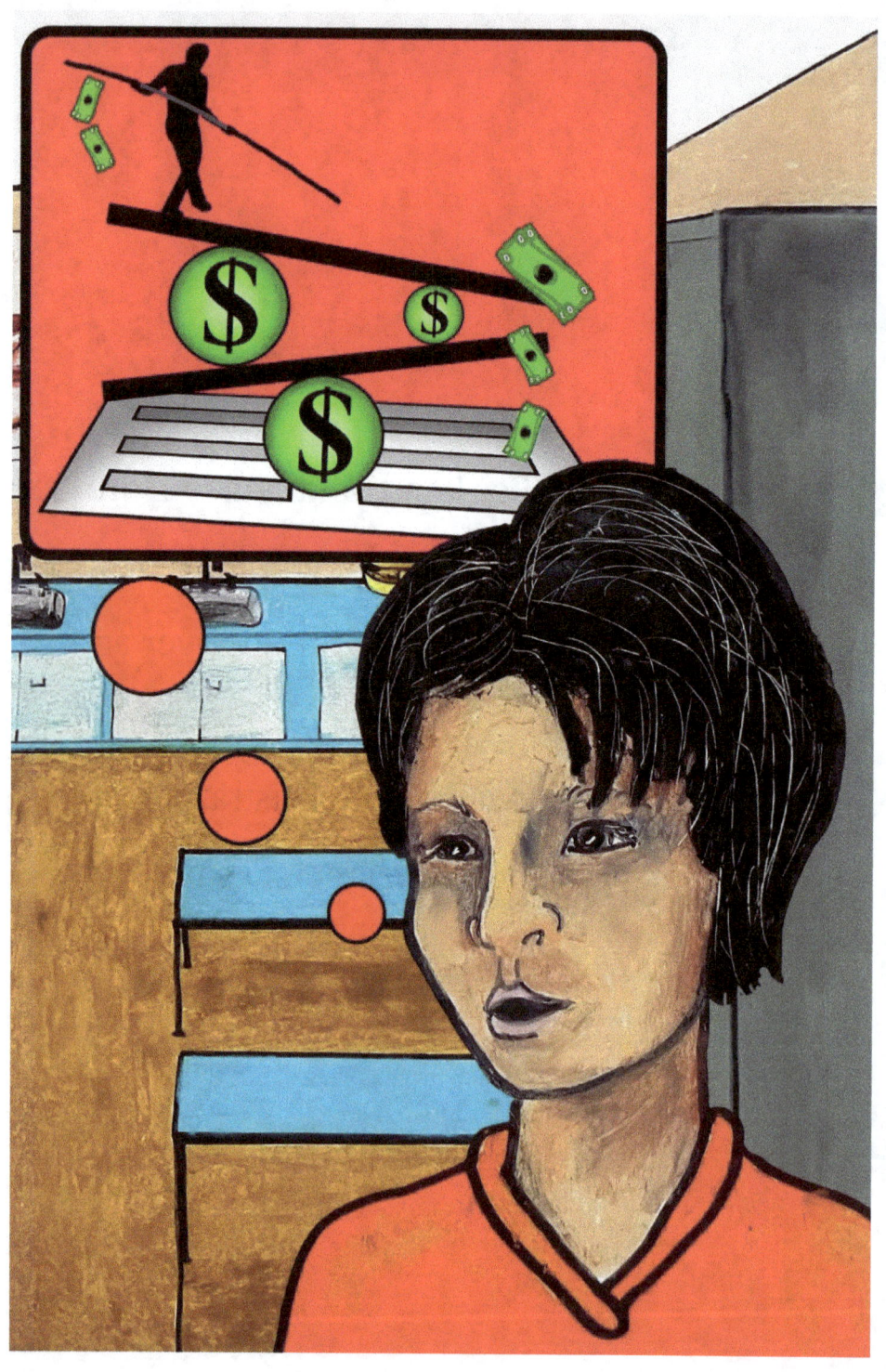

Kenji raises his hand, and Nurse Dorothea calls on him to talk. "My mom lost her job a while back, and we were financially unstable. It really affected me because I couldn't buy all the clothes I wanted. I couldn't buy all my favorite snacks, and we had to skip eating at restaurants. It made me angry that we were in that situation and couldn't do what we wanted."

"Financial difficulties can disturb a person's mental well-being, so that is another reason we should stay lifelong learners and continue increasing our skill set so that we can easily adapt and get new jobs if our old job goes away," says Nurse Dorothea.

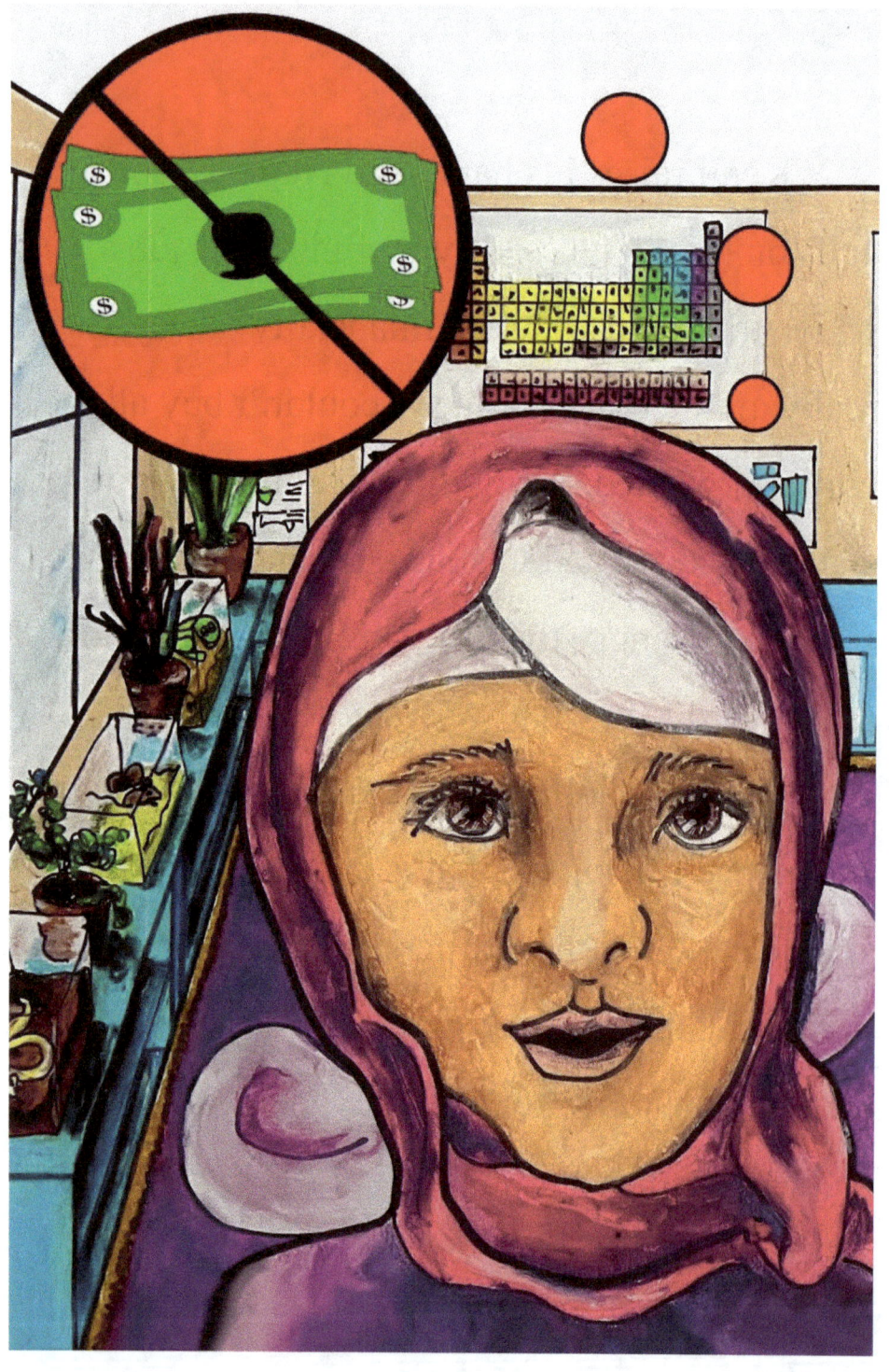

Fatima raises her hand, and Nurse Dorothea calls on her to talk. "My parents talk about the debt they have and I know that is the reason we can't take vacations every year. It makes me angry to see my parents struggle."

"Having some debt may be good for different reasons, but when a family's debt load is too much, it can affect everyone's lifestyle. We should all use caution about how much debt we take on. People can get advice from financial advisors to guide their decisions so that the family is financially healthy," says Nurse Dorothea.

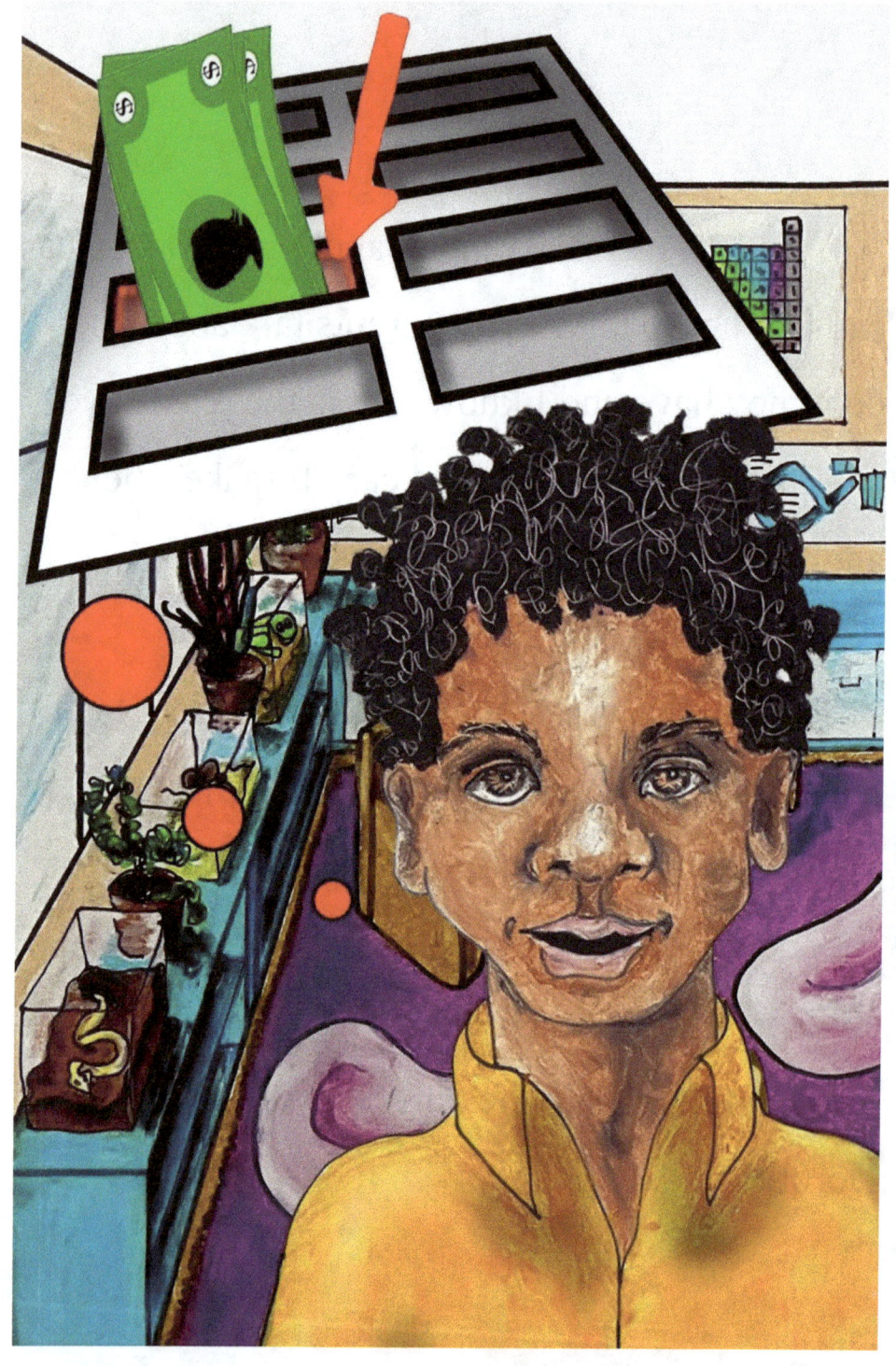

Amari raises his hand, and Nurse Dorothea calls on him to talk. "I get angry when I feel like I've wasted my money. I don't have a lot of money to spend on fun things, so when I go see a bad movie in the movie theaters, I feel I've wasted my money and can't get a refund. It makes me angry about the money I spent when I could have done something else like bowling."

"It's important to stay focused on doing things as a family or with friends to connect and have better relationships with them instead of doing things with family and friends just to do things. We should do things so that our relationships become stronger and not worry about what was spent or used to develop the relationship," says Nurse Dorothea.

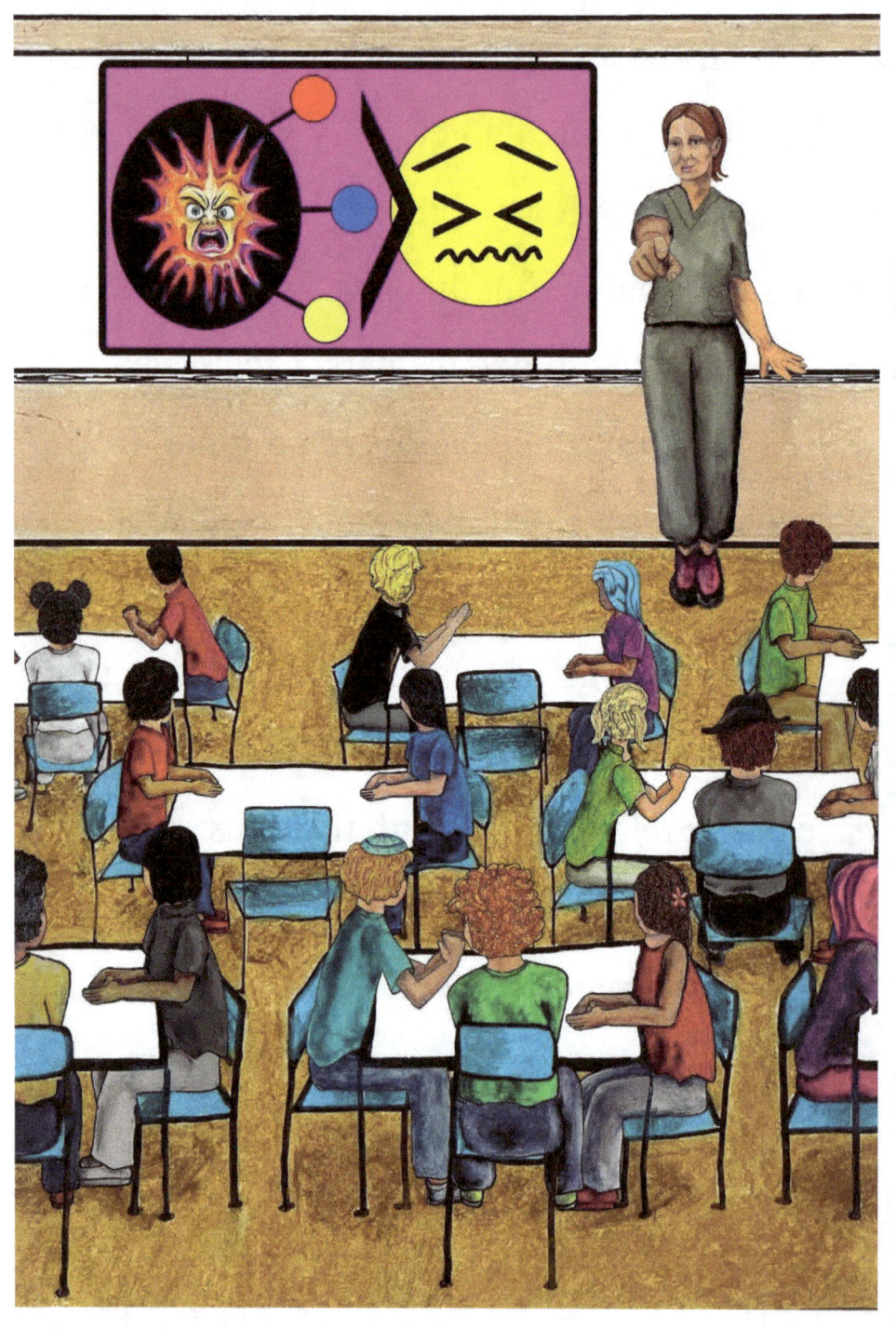

"Anger can cause us to be impulsive and do things we regret. It could be harsh words that were said to someone, which may have broken a relationship, or acting out in violence that leads to property destruction, which could cause legal problems. Worse, anger could cause us to hurt someone, including ourselves. Let's take some time to discuss some things you may have done out of anger that you later regretted. Let's talk with each other now."

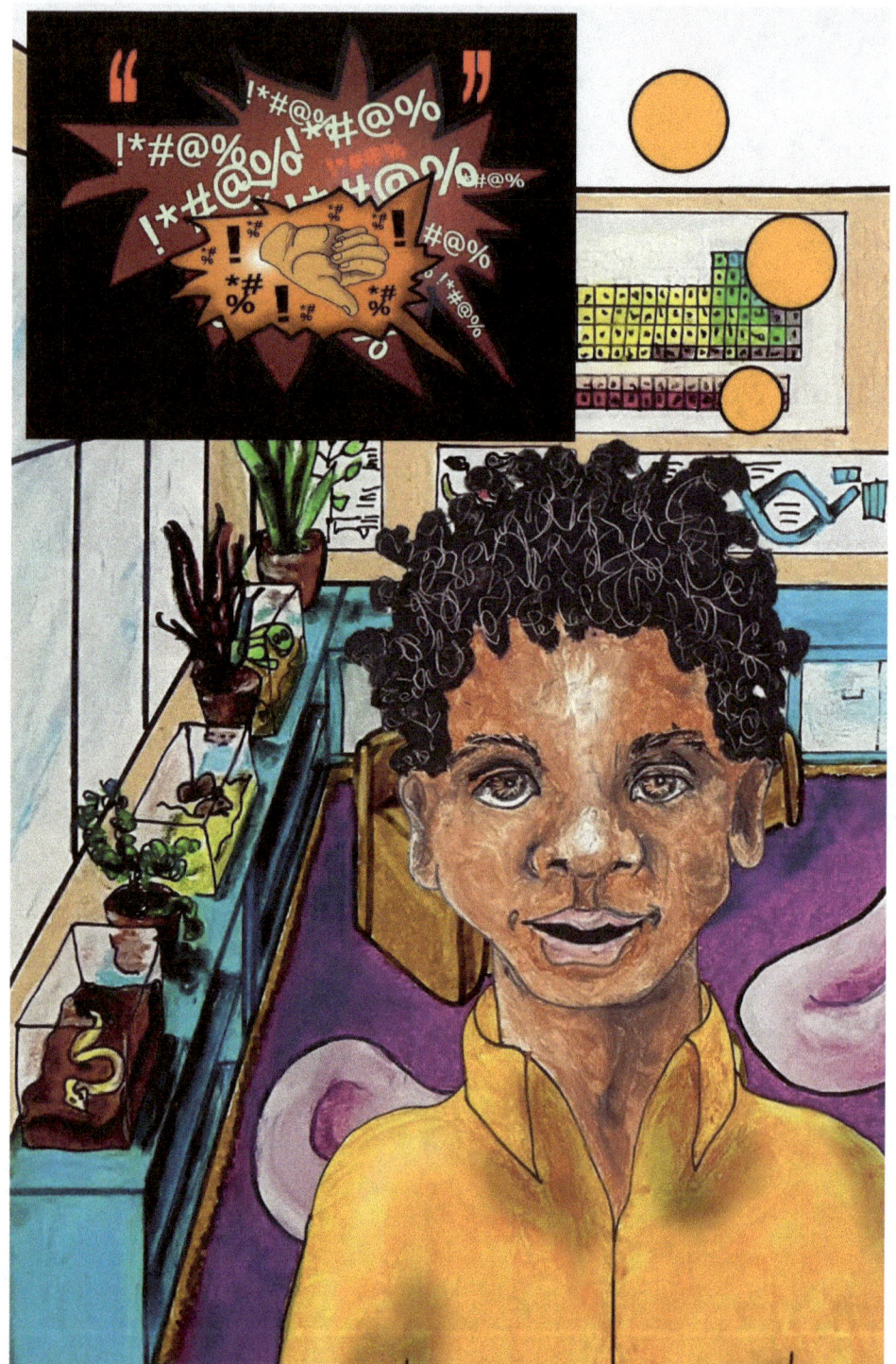

Amari raises his hand, and Nurse Dorothea calls on him to talk. "Once, when someone was being disrespectful to me, I got angry and started saying rude and disrespectful things back. I tried to say meaner things than they were saying to me. Later, I regretted it because I think I went too far."

"Anger can cause things to escalate and turn a bad situation into something much worse, so that is why we need to learn to manage our anger," says Nurse Dorothea.

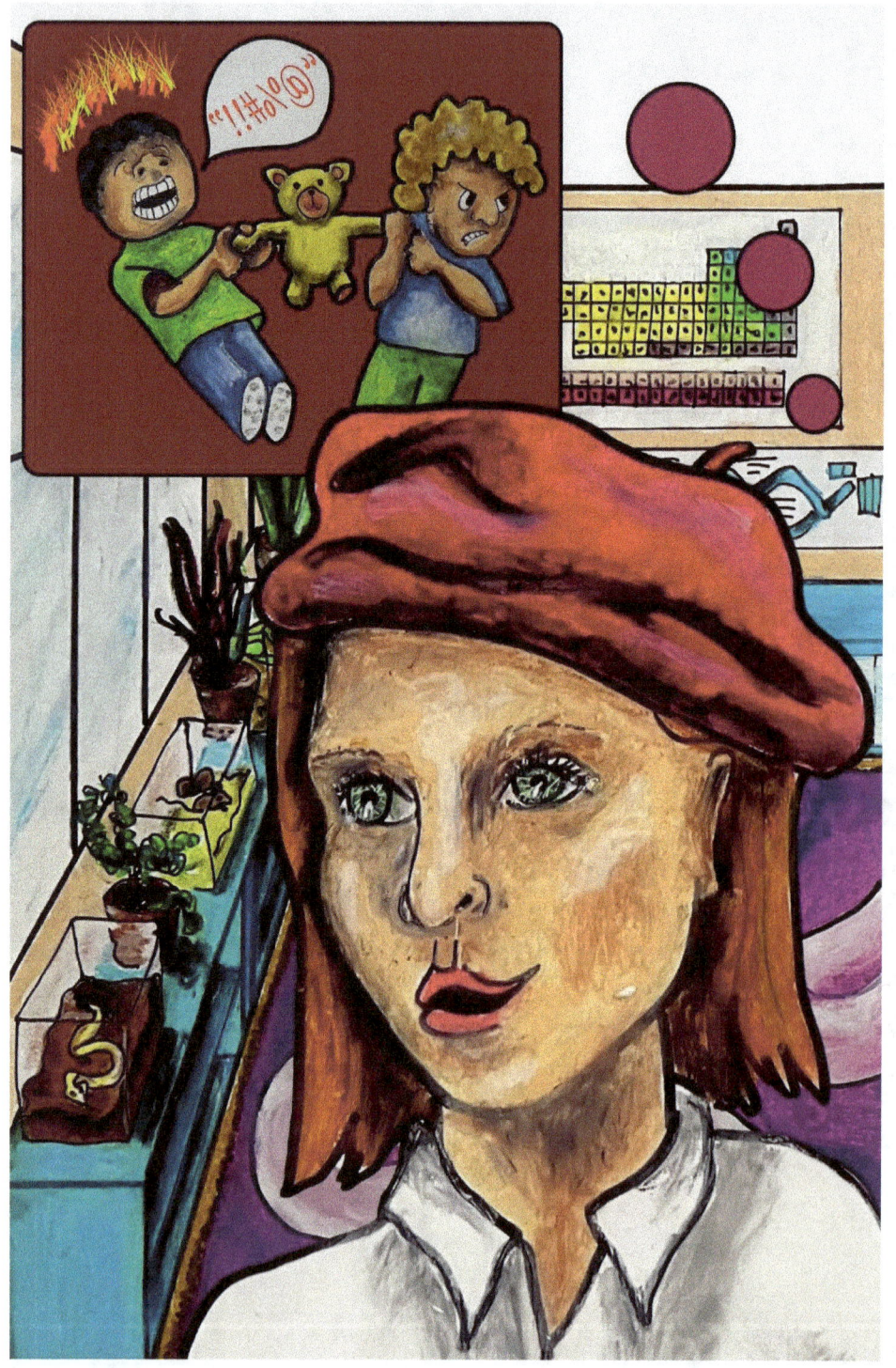

Marie raises her hand, and Nurse Dorothea calls on her to talk. "When I was younger, I would get angry with my brother, and we would fight over toys. There were times that we broke the toy, and then both of us got sad."

"Anger that turns into fighting can easily lead to damaged property. It is good to control your anger early in life so that you don't destroy property in the future and regret it along with having legal problems," says Nurse Dorothea.

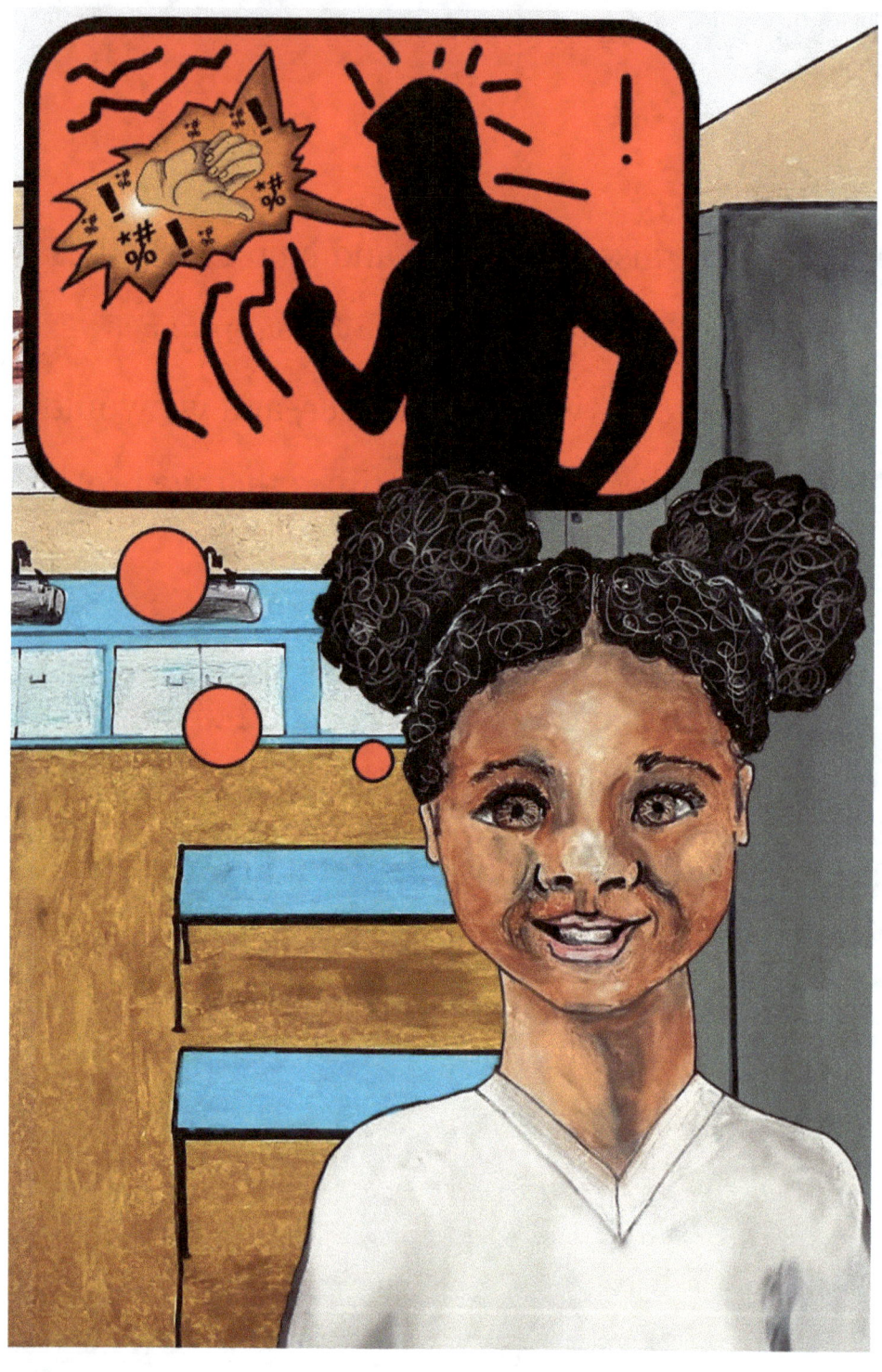

Amisha raises her hand, and Nurse Dorothea calls on her to talk. "I've gotten into arguments with my parents, and once, I said some really hurtful things to them. I said I wish they weren't my parents. Later, I heard my dad crying because of it. I felt really bad and couldn't take it back. I have a good relationship with my parents and don't want to hurt them like that again."

"Sometimes, we can burn bridges with our words to the extent that some people will choose to stop helping us. Think before you speak to avoid regret," says Nurse Dorothea.

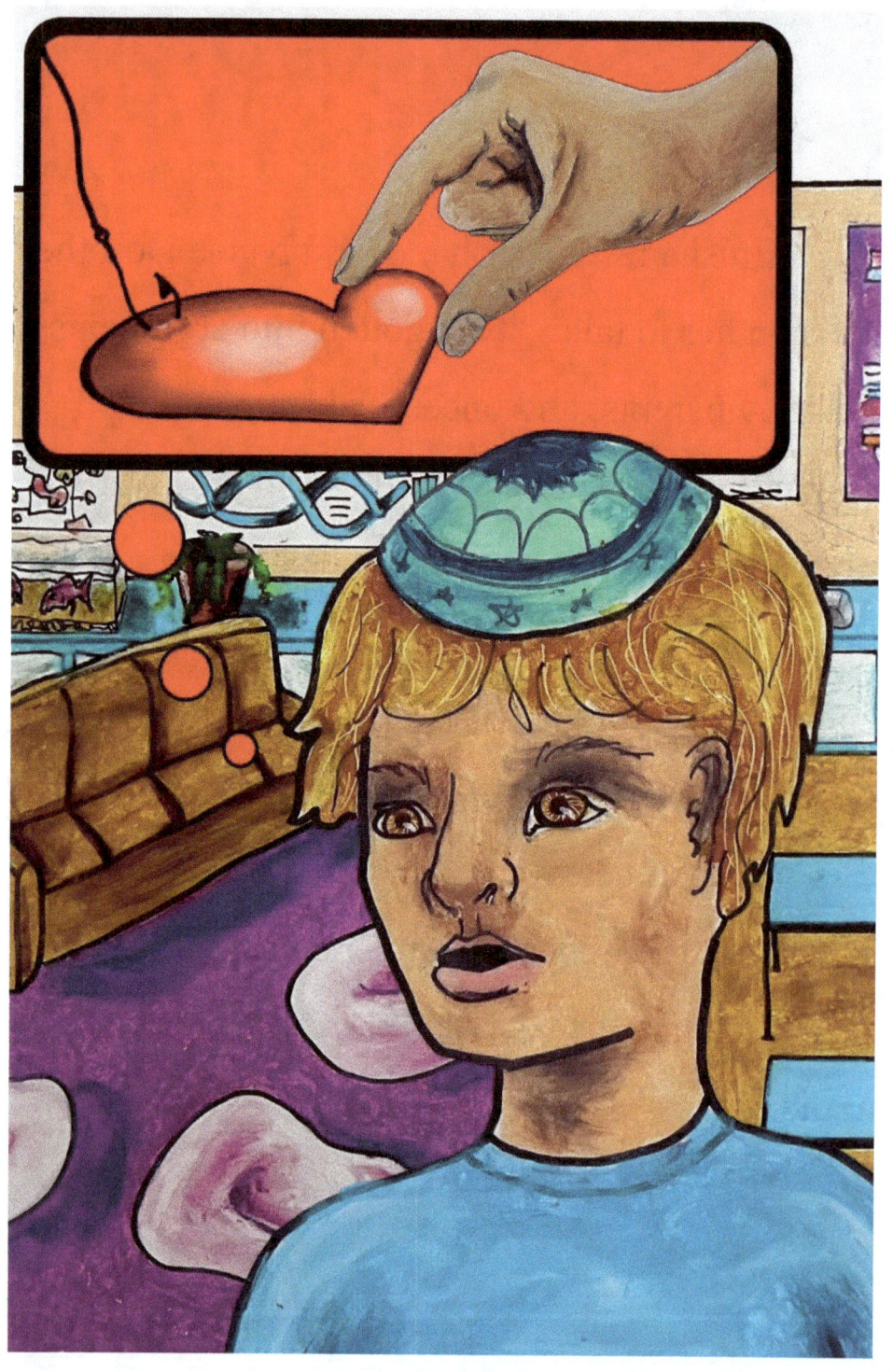

Levi raises his hand, and Nurse Dorothea calls on him to talk. "I acted out of revenge once when I thought my heart was being played with. I helped cause some of my ex-partner's friends to not like her anymore, and it was a mean thing to do. I wish I wouldn't have done that."

"Acting out of anger can cause regretful actions. Regret can disrupt our mental well-being," says Nurse Dorothea.

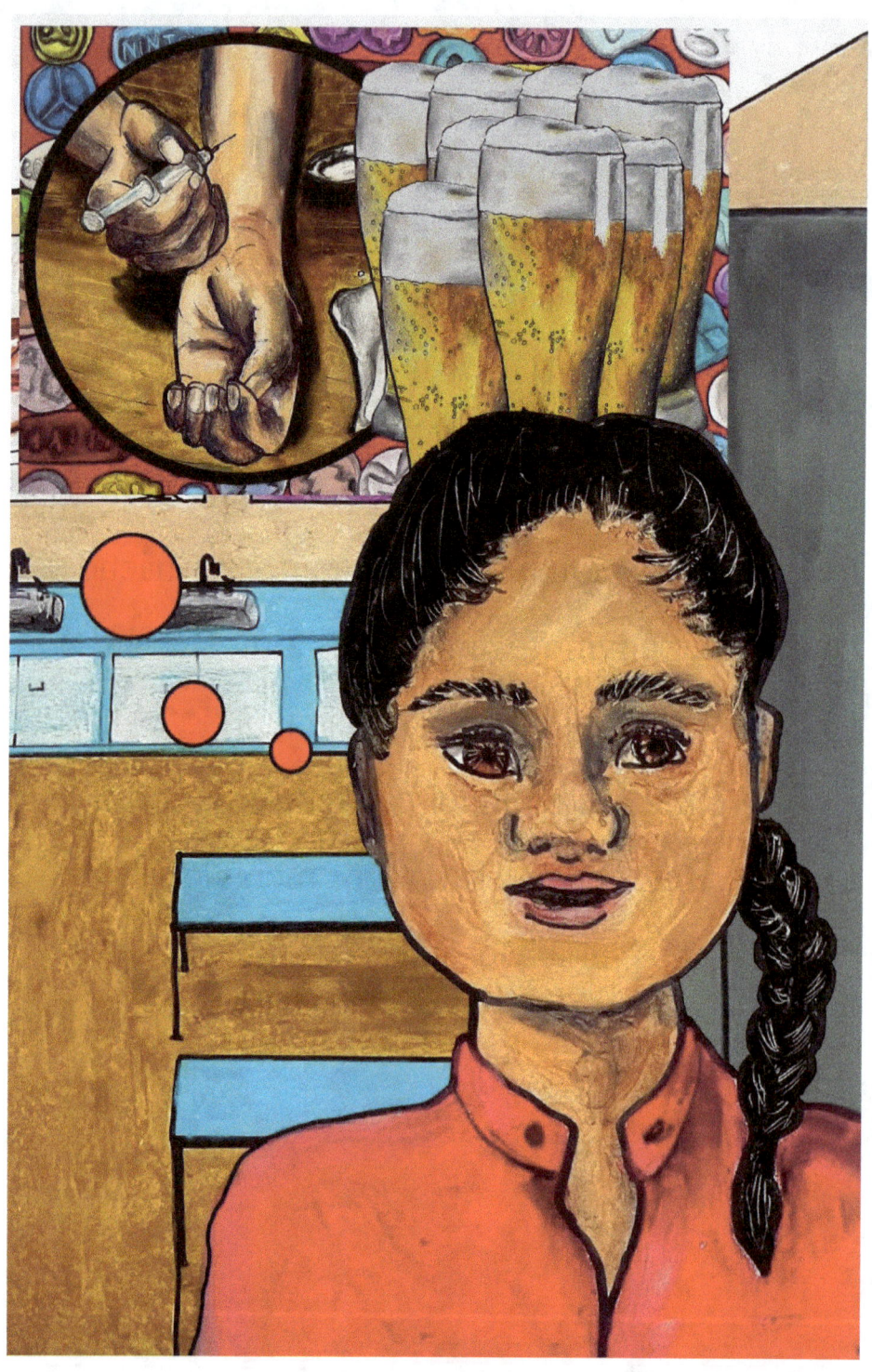

Pia raises her hand, and Nurse Dorothea calls on her to talk. "I saw my brother get very angry at my parents, and then he went to his room. When my parents checked on him later, he was abusing some drugs. I've seen how anger can lead to substance abuse, and it can destroy someone's life."

"Substance abuse is a temporary fix to a problem since it causes the person to have better feelings temporarily, so they can avoid their problems or emotions. People should get therapy or engage in other healthy coping skills when they get angry if they are considering substance abuse," says Nurse Dorothea.

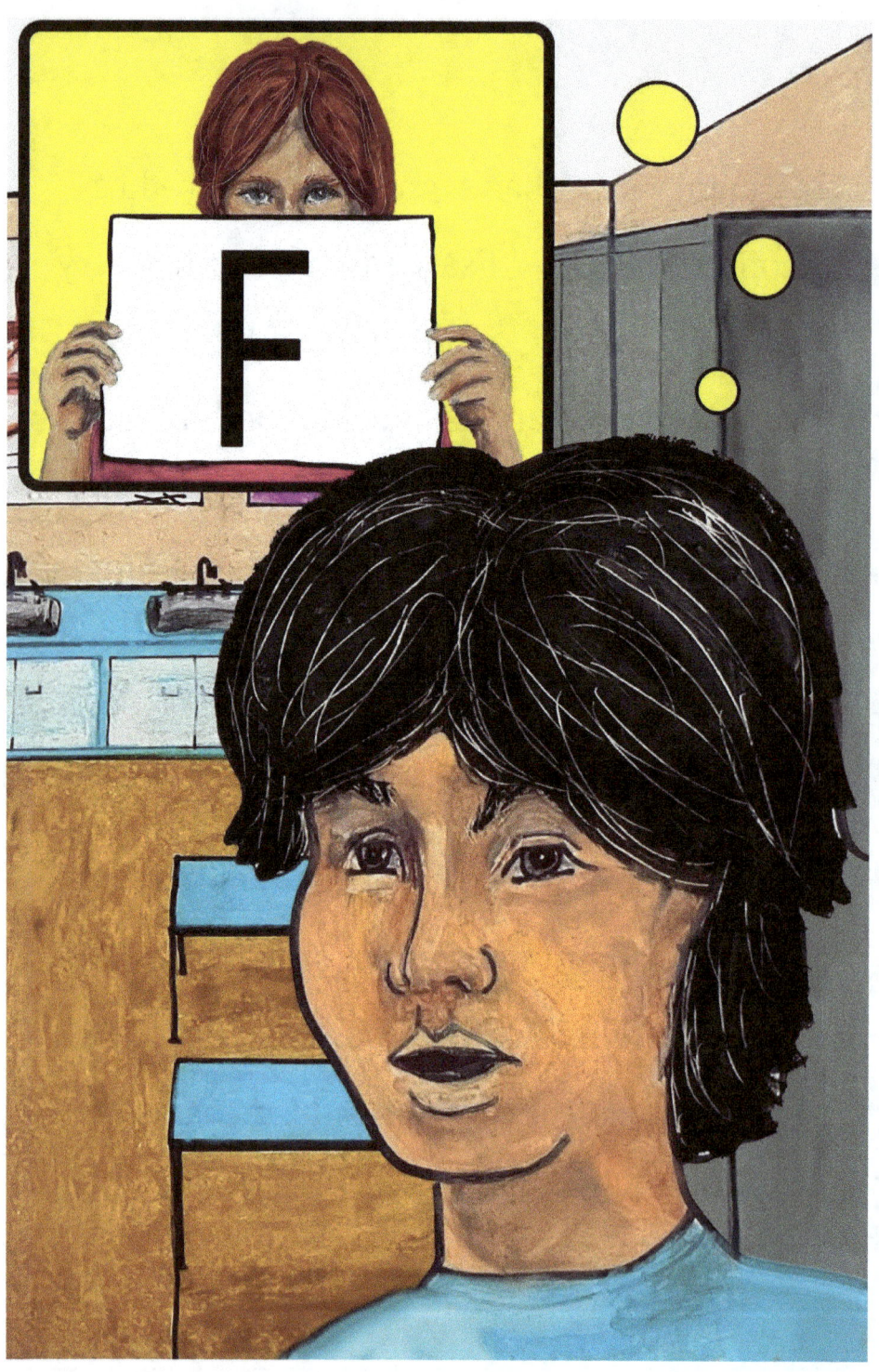

Ji Ho raises his hand, and Nurse Dorothea calls on him to talk. "I got poor grades one semester and got very angry at my teacher. I wanted to say something mean but held it back. That night, I thought about it more and realized it was my fault I got a bad grade, because I didn't study for any of the exams. I felt dumb because I wanted to act out against my teacher and also because I realized I was lazy."

"Anger at yourself can lead a person to low self-esteem so we should face our anger toward ourselves and turn it into productivity by developing new skills and abilities so that we can increase our self-confidence," says Nurse Dorothea.

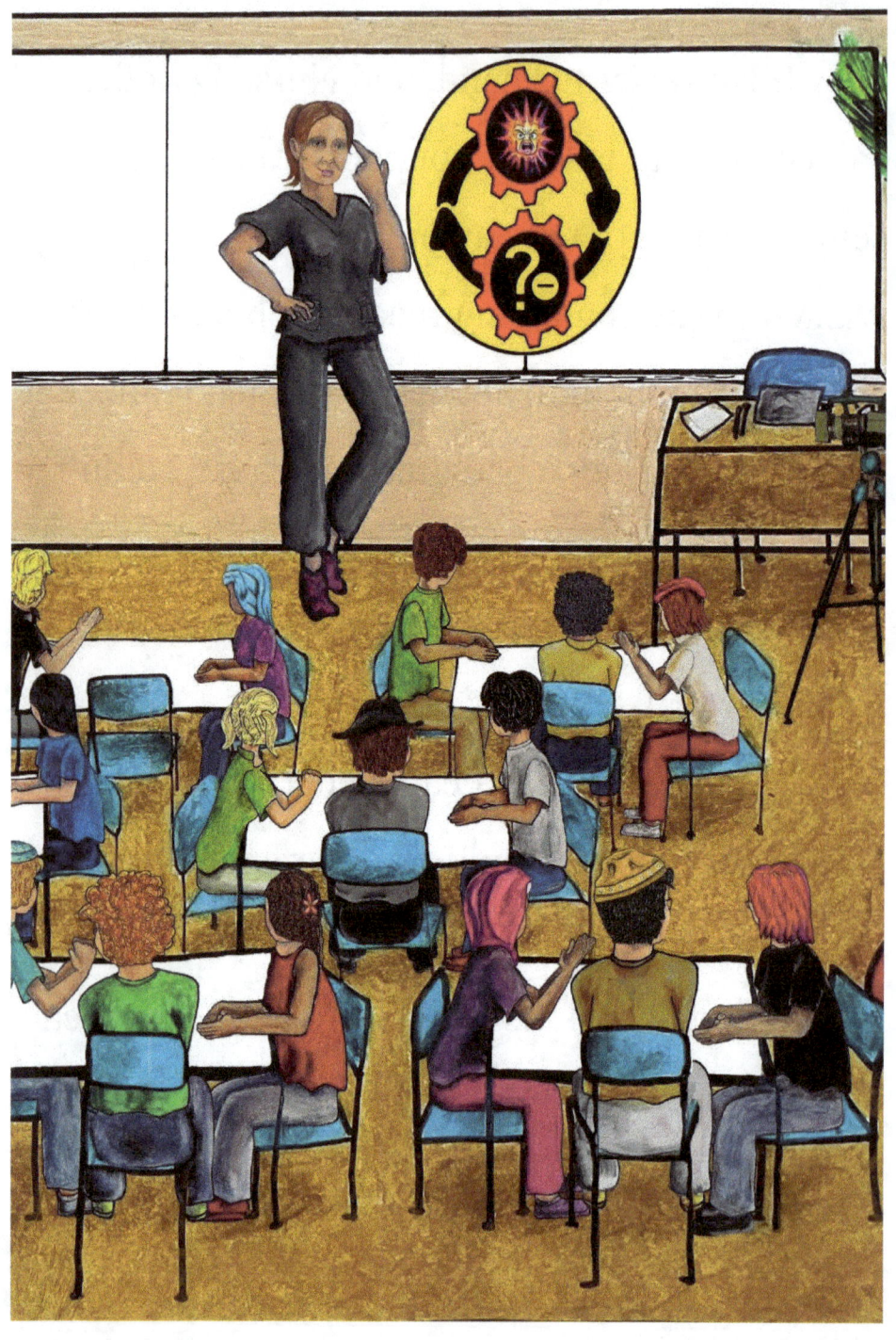

"Anger can impact a lot of things like relationships, employment, finances, health, and more. I'd like you all to discuss something that anger has negatively impacted in your life in the long term. Share with those around you or write in your journal now, please."

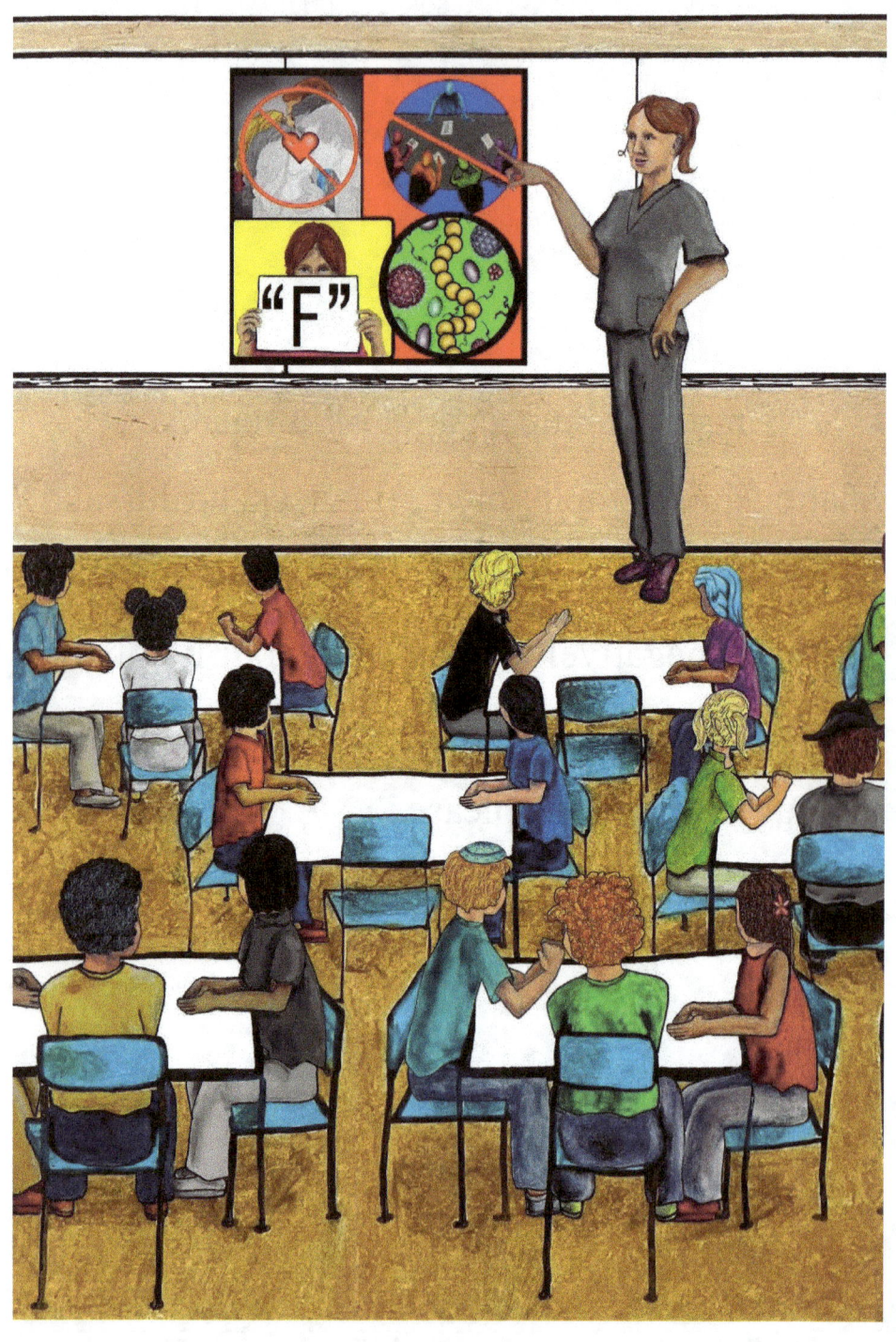

After a time for discussion, Nurse Dorothea continues, "Destructive behaviors in words and deeds can lead a person to lose a job, lose friendships, lose a marriage, lose a relationship with different family members, get poor grades in school, get in trouble with law enforcement, and reduce self-respect. Anger can even lead a body into certain diseases due to the associated stress. I'm not saying that we should never get angry, but we should learn to manage our anger so that it is productive for our lives as a whole instead of simply destroying things. Anger is part of the human existence and is seen in the animal world. Some would even say that mother nature gets angry as seen with destructive storms and natural disasters. Let's learn to harness our anger like a wild horse, so that it can be tamed and used to support society."

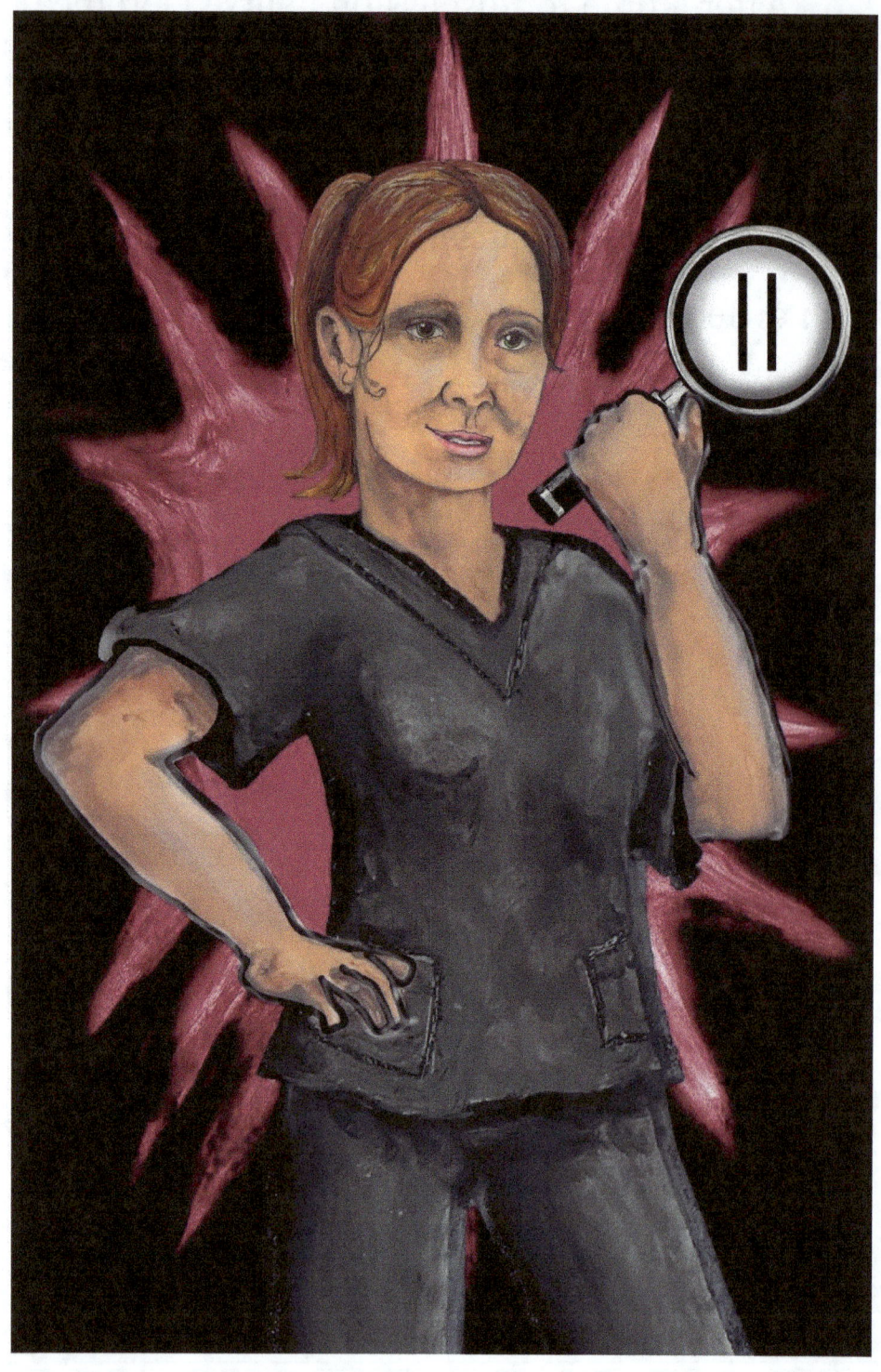

"We have gone over a lot of things that may have surfaced some unpleasant feelings, so let's take a short break and refresh ourselves. Those of you watching the video or reading the book, continue the lesson whenever you are ready. We'll see each other shortly."

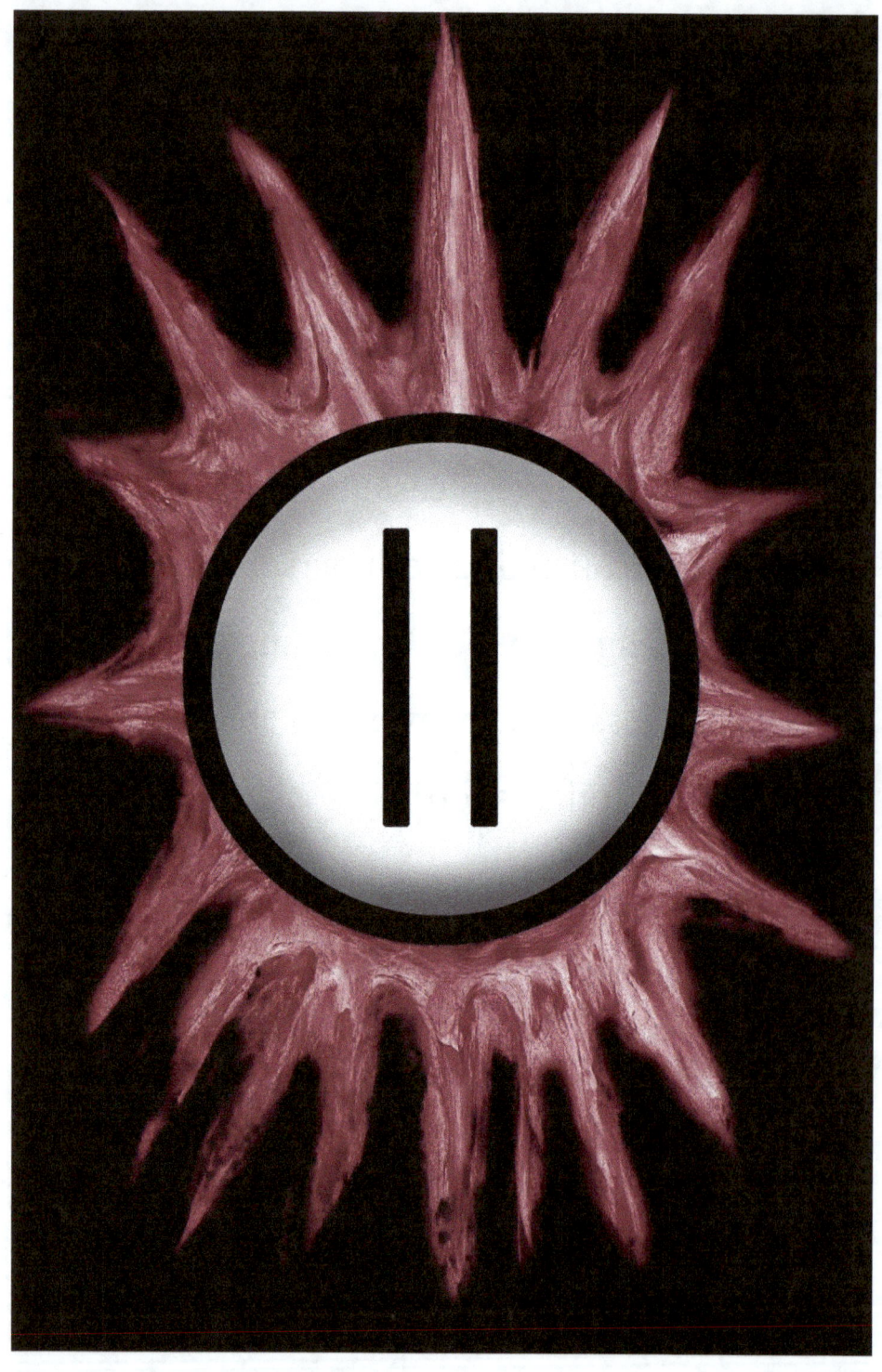

Part 2

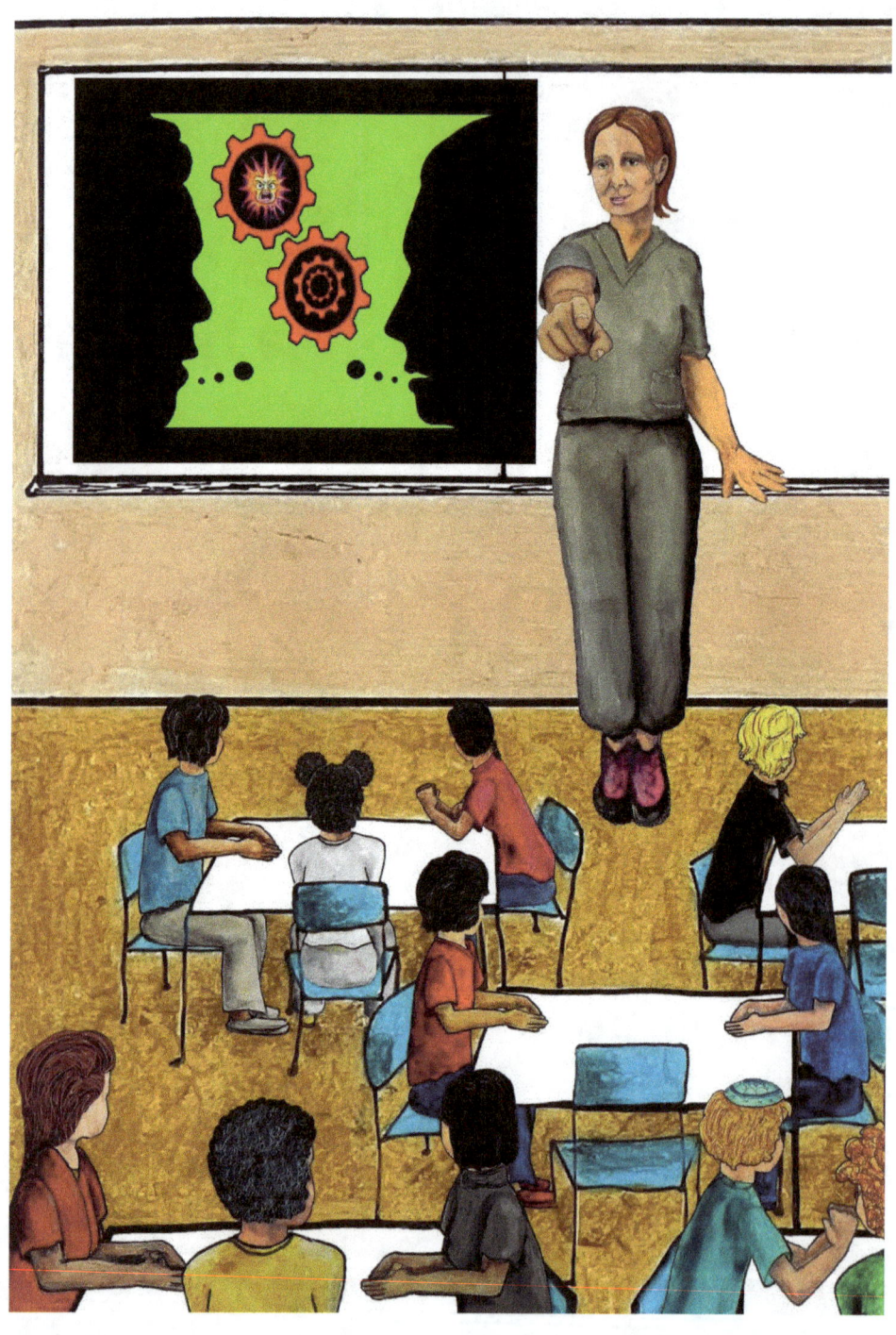

"Welcome back, everyone! People cope with anger in many ways, some healthy and some unhealthy. Some use anger to destroy their lives and those around themselves, while others use anger to strengthen their lives into better ones. I'd like us all to take some time to think about the positive or constructive things we have done to deal with our anger. Anger is a powerful force, and we can use that energy to make things better. Share your tips or experiences with those around you, and we'll discuss as a class. If you are doing this class by yourself, go ahead and write in your journal."

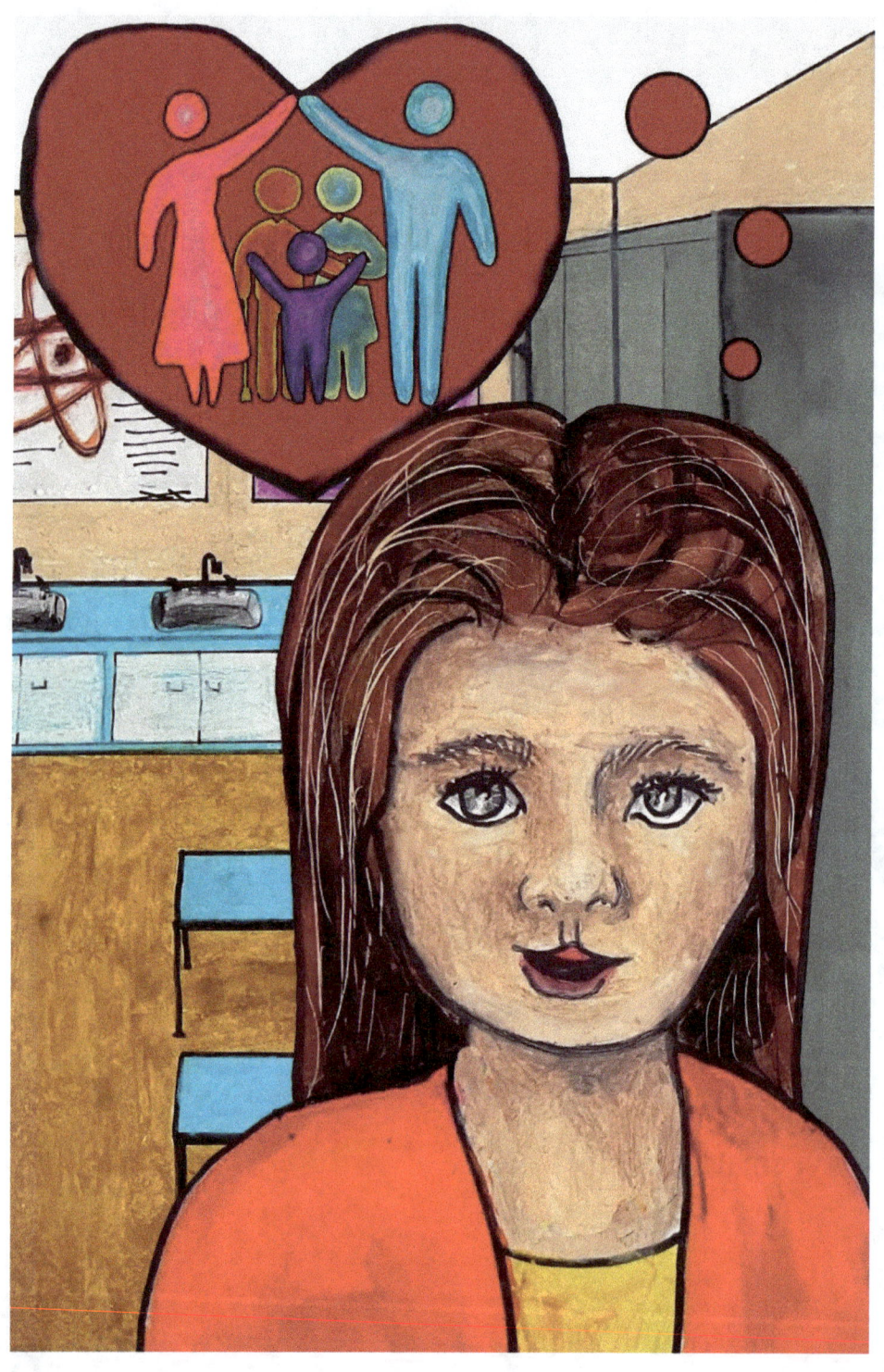

Awira raises her hand, and Nurse Dorothea calls on her to talk. "I went through some difficult things with my parents and became angry at them. I was sitting in my room one day, angry, and I realized it was pointless if I did nothing about why I was angry. I got up and went to my parents to talk about the things that were making me angry. I chose to use my anger as a sign to get me to communicate more with those I was angry with. Talking more with my parents has really helped our relationship, and we are at a lot closer now. Anger can show an area of weakness, and I chose to strengthen my communication skills."

"That is beautiful that you used anger to show you where you could improve and make things better. Good job!" says Nurse Dorothea.

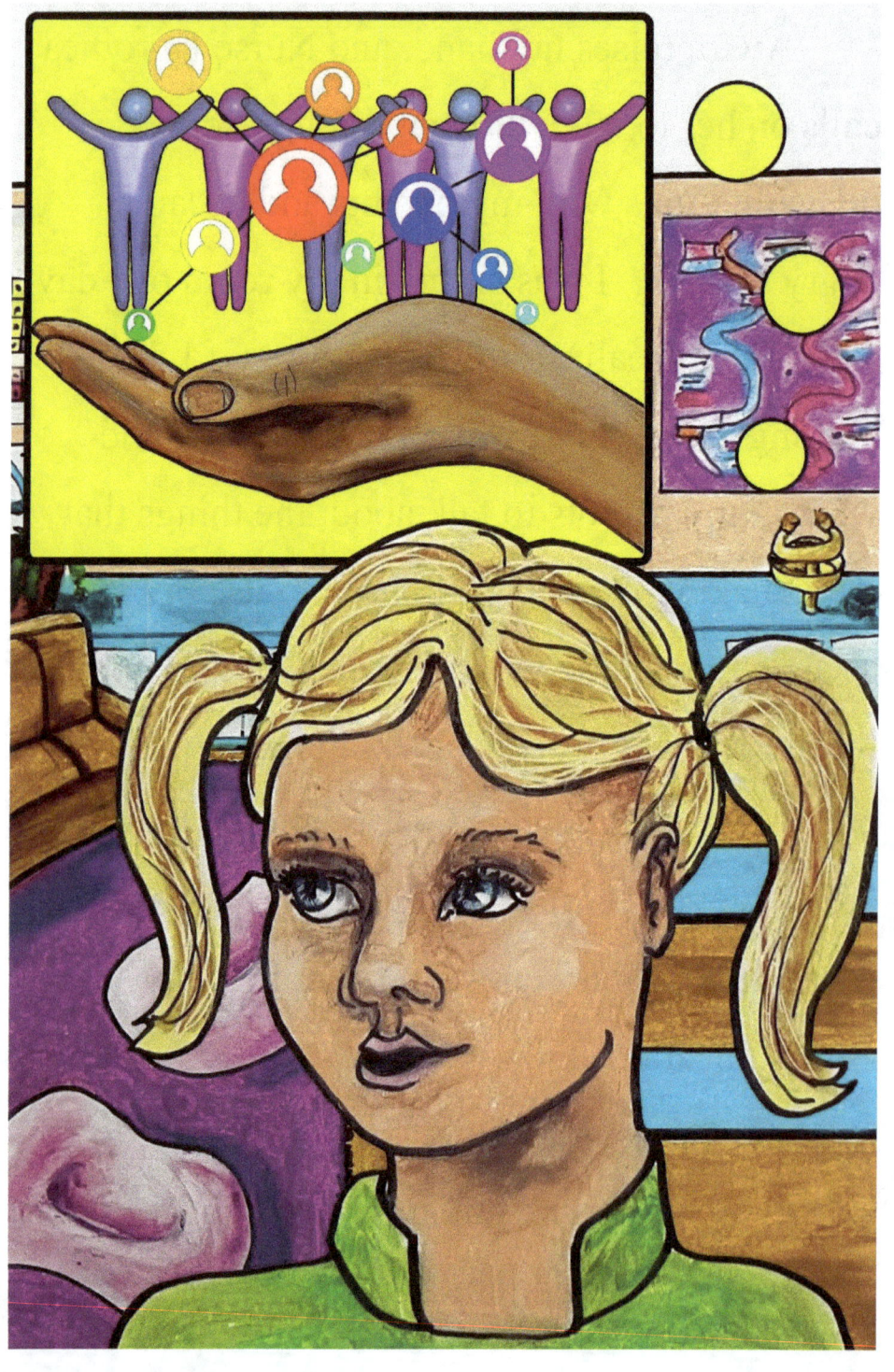

Frida raises her hand, and Nurse Dorothea calls on her to talk. "I was lonely, and that made me frustrated. I felt like no one cared. I was also sitting in my room alone one day and realized that maybe I was lonely because of my not trying to socialize. From that day on, I decided I would try to make a new friend each month. I have been more outgoing and realize that socializing is a skill, and we all need to develop our social skills. I now have many friends from all types of backgrounds who have interests in many things, which helps me to do different activities every month. Friends are fun!"

"Developing friendships are important since sometimes you only make it through a hard part in your life when you have a strong friend network," says Nurse Dorothea.

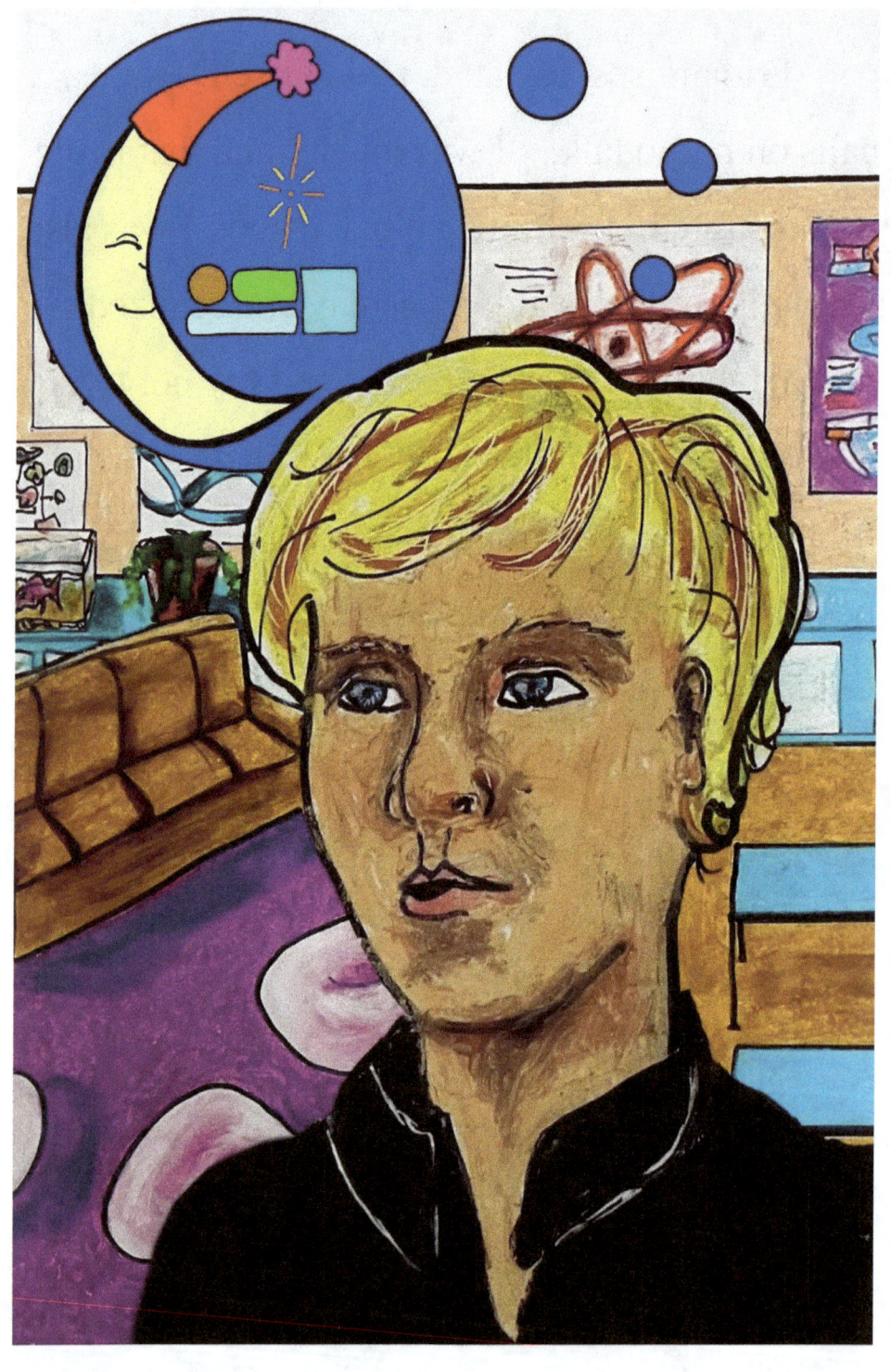

Dimitry raises his hand, and Nurse Dorothea calls on him to talk. "I would get frustrated with things at school, and one morning I woke up and realized my frustration wasn't there. I realized I had gone to bed early that night and had gotten really good sleep. It hit me that getting good sleep was a key to good management of emotions, so now I go to sleep kind of early every night. It helps me get a good night's rest. I have a sleep routine like getting a shower, brushing my teeth, and then listening to 15 minutes of relaxing music before I close my eyes. Good sleep has really helped me."

"Good sleep can help not only with emotions, but also with having good health," says Nurse Dorothea.

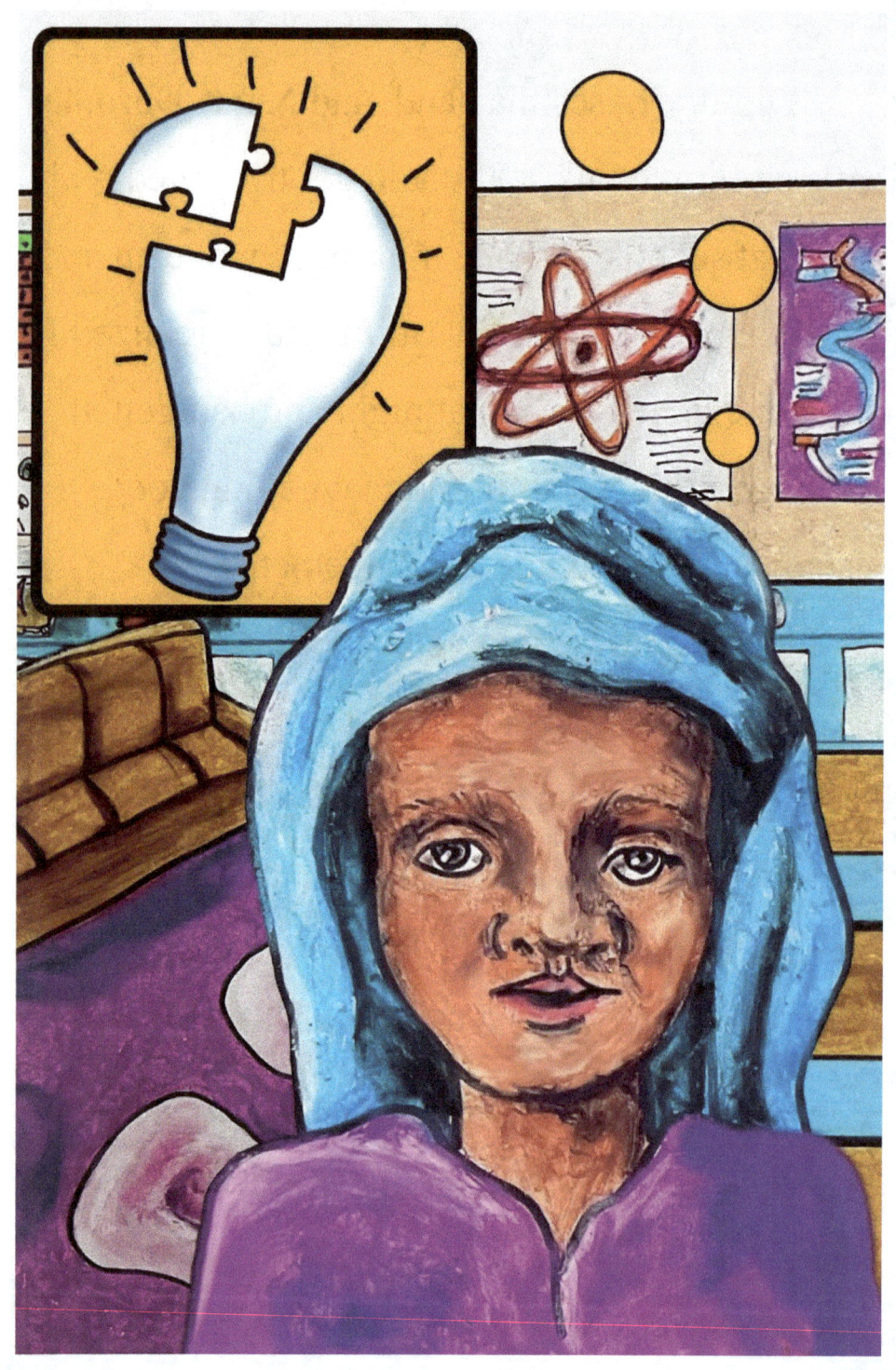

Yuliana raises her hand, and Nurse Dorothea calls on her to talk. "I was angry about tasks not being completed, so I decided to use my anger to focus and become a problem solver. Now, when I get angry about something, I choose to see it as a problem to solve and will talk to different people to get ideas on how to solve the problem. Anger has pointed me in the right direction since I allowed it to."

"That's excellent that you used anger to motivate you to problem solve and to increase your communication skills. Using our emotions to better our lives is very important and the sooner we start doing that, the better. It's never too late to start, since adapting and changing will be a good role model for others to see that it's never too late to start improving your life," says Nurse Dorothea.

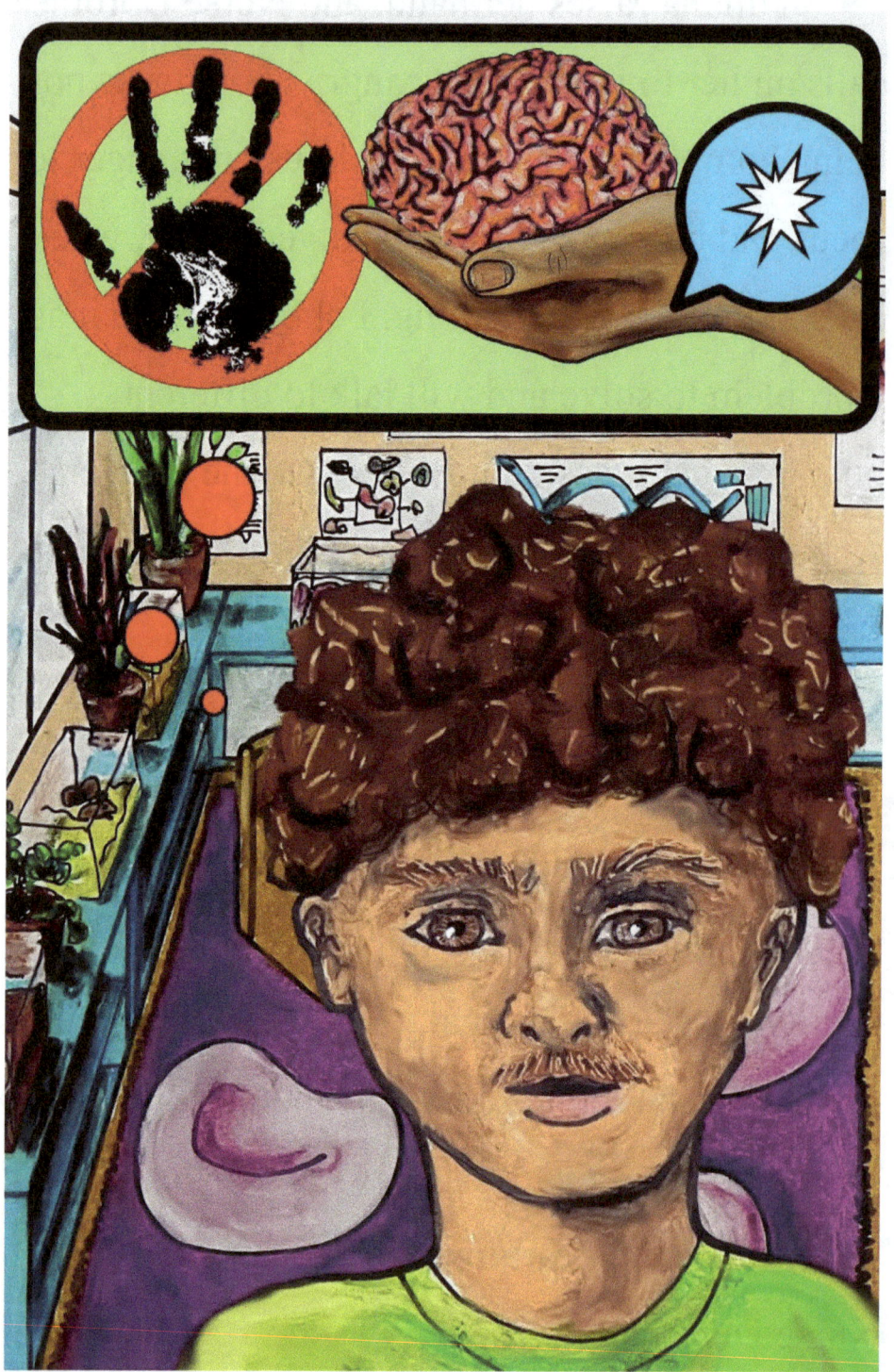

Gustavo raises his hand, and Nurse Dorothea calls on him to talk. "Since I've said some things that I regretted out of my anger, I choose to use anger as a sign that I need to slow down and think before speaking. One thing that I will do is write out a letter in anger towards the person with whom I am having issues. This helps get all my thoughts out. Later, I will sit down and read what I wrote and try to see if everything I was thinking was valid, and if I should be angry about the situation. This helps me gain different perspectives and gives some space between me and the other person."

"Journaling is a great healthy coping skill. Great use of your resources!" says Nurse Dorothea.

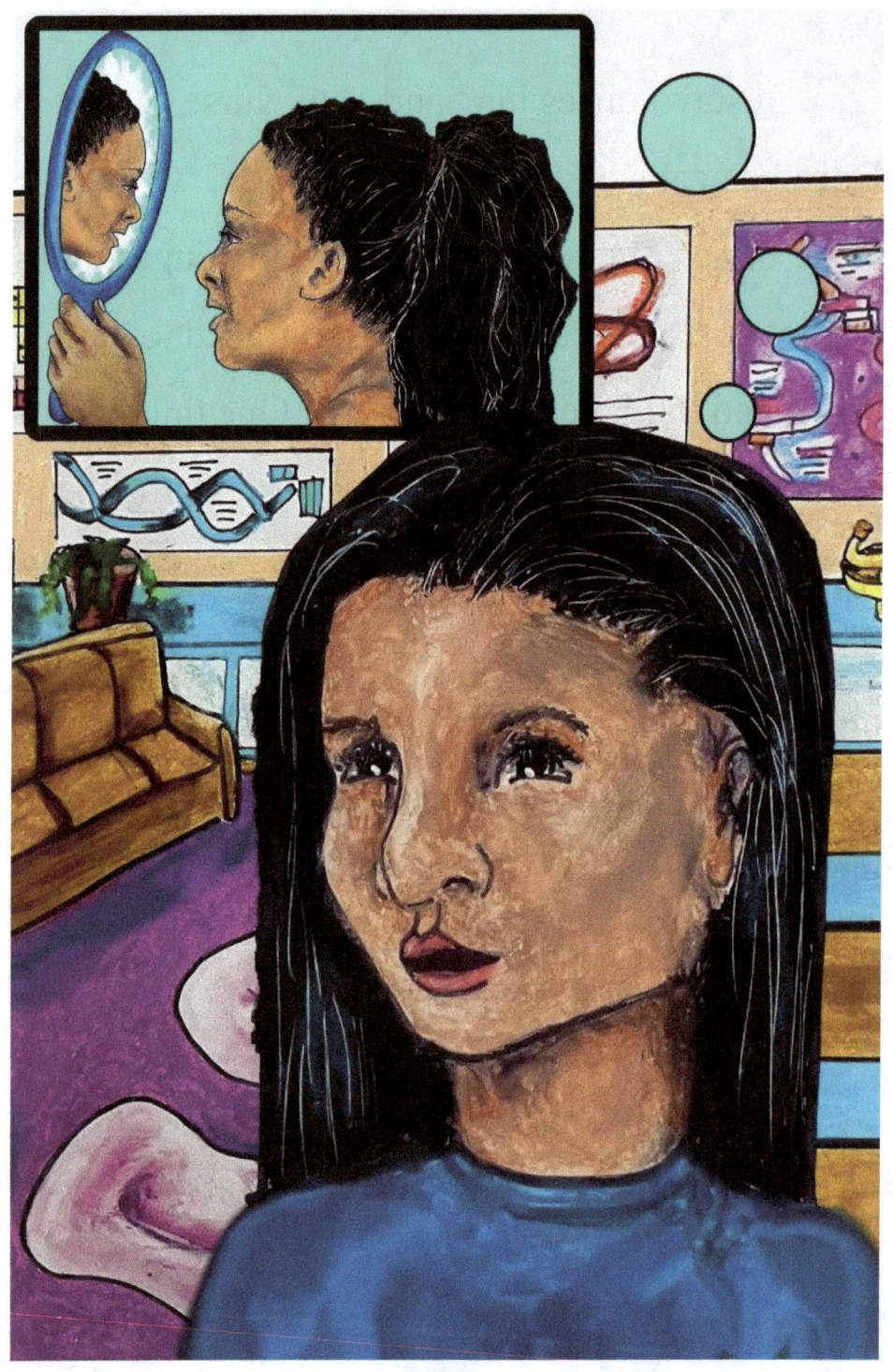

Diwa raises her hand, and Nurse Dorothea calls on her to talk. "Once I got angry and did some things I regretted. I vowed not to let myself do something like that again. I choose to use anger as a signal that I need to do some self-reflection to see if I was the cause of my anger, or if I caused the other person to do something which then led to my anger. I have learned about myself and have grown as a person since I started doing that."

"Insight about oneself and learning why we do the things that we do is key for a successful mental health journey through life. Seek to know yourself," says Nurse Dorothea.

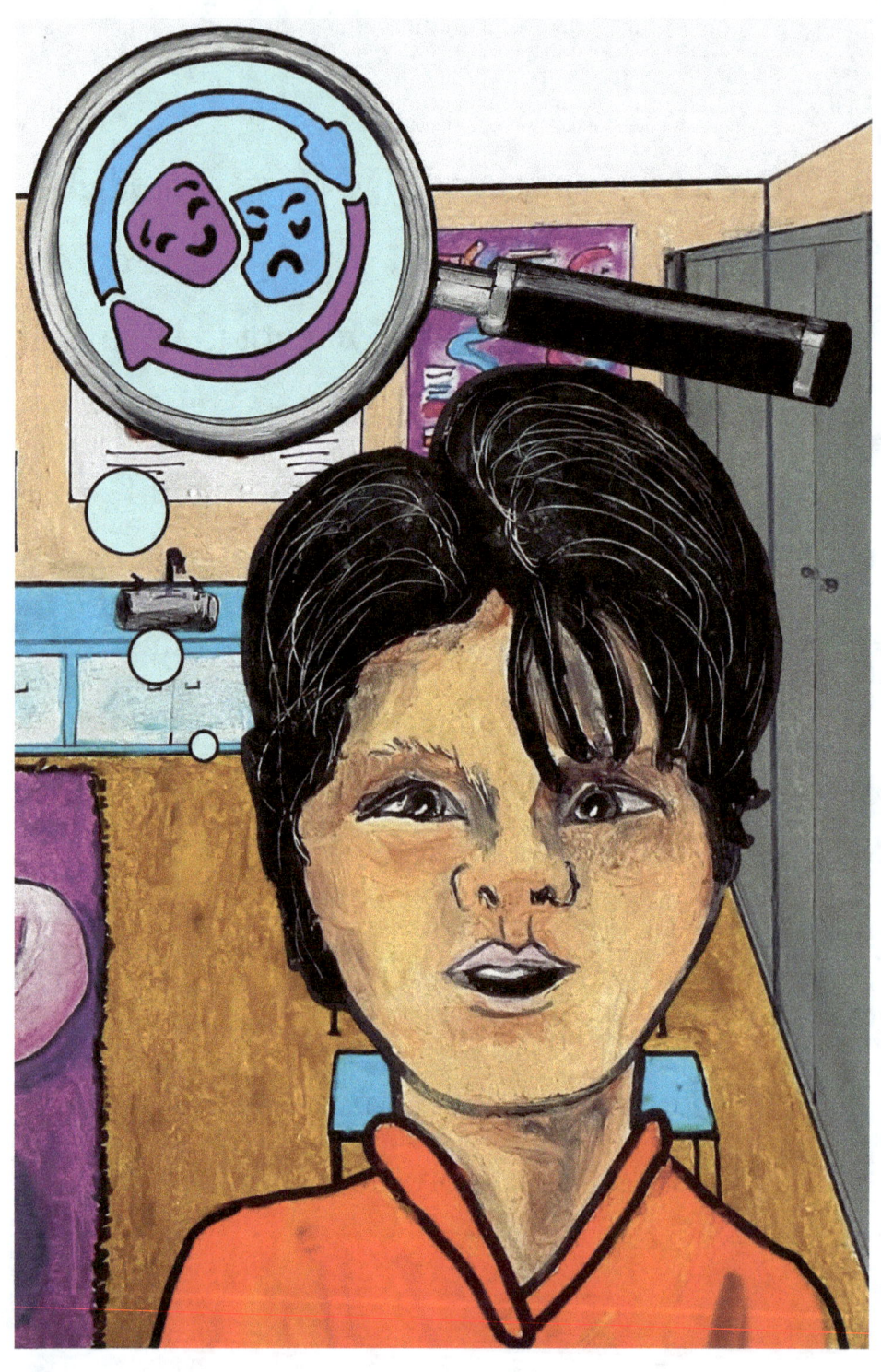

Kenji raises his hand, and Nurse Dorothea calls on him to talk. "Anger sometimes scares me, because I'm not sure how destructive I could become. I use my anger as a sign that I need to be more aware and mindful of my emotions. I need to understand my triggers. I need to understand how I want to automatically reply to things. I think being more aware of my emotions has helped me manage them better, although I still have work to do."

"Emotional awareness can lead to greater emotional intelligence, and we all have more work to do," says Nurse Dorothea.

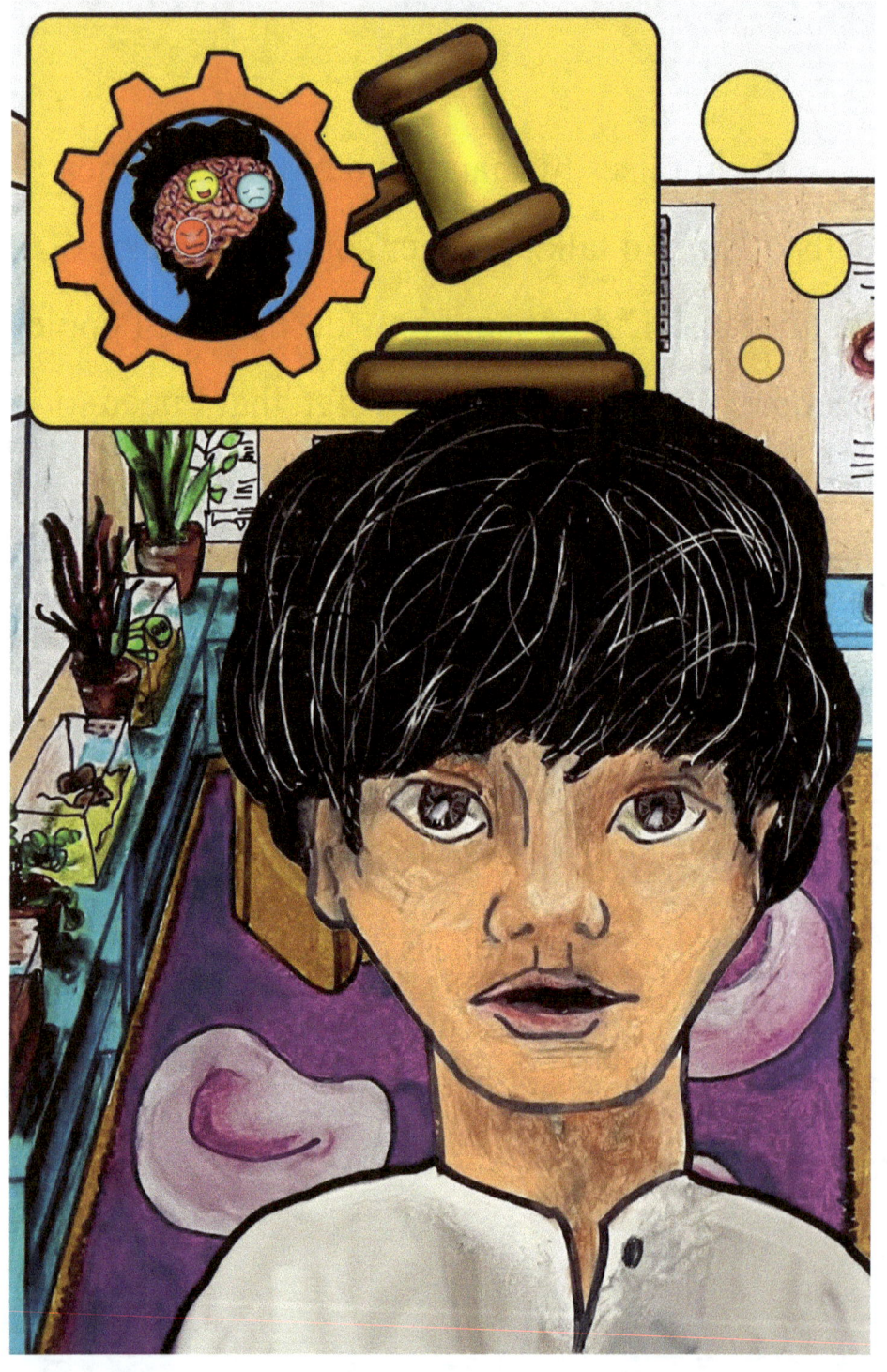

Antonio raises his hand, and Nurse Dorothea calls on him to talk. "Because my anger can be so strong, I realized years ago that I need to regulate my emotions. I need to live a balanced life. I need to seek to live in peaceful equilibrium, so that I can calmly deal with the negative things in my life. It's hard, but I strive for that every day."

"Emotional homeostasis is hard to do since we are so complicated, and the world we live in is complex. Learning to stay at peace and to return to peace after something disrupts your mental equilibrium is an important skill and can help you respond to emotional things with tranquility. We achieve that skill by using many different coping skills and using the right coping skill for the right situation at the right time," says Nurse Dorothea.

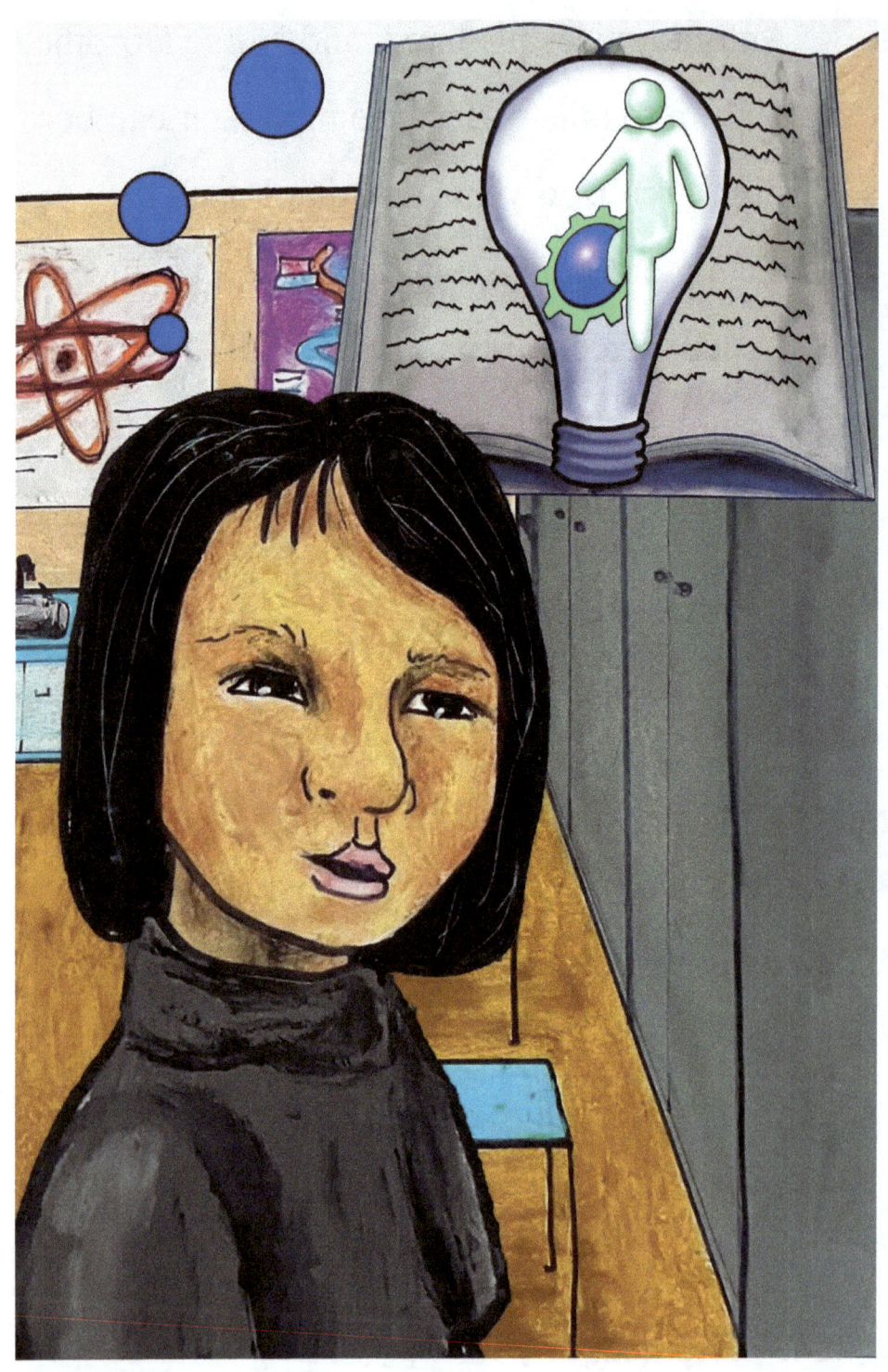

Lian raises her hand, and Nurse Dorothea calls on her to talk. "I use my anger to give me the energy to be assertive. I say what I mean, mean what I say, and don't say it mean."

"Assertiveness is an important part of effective communication," says Nurse Dorothea.

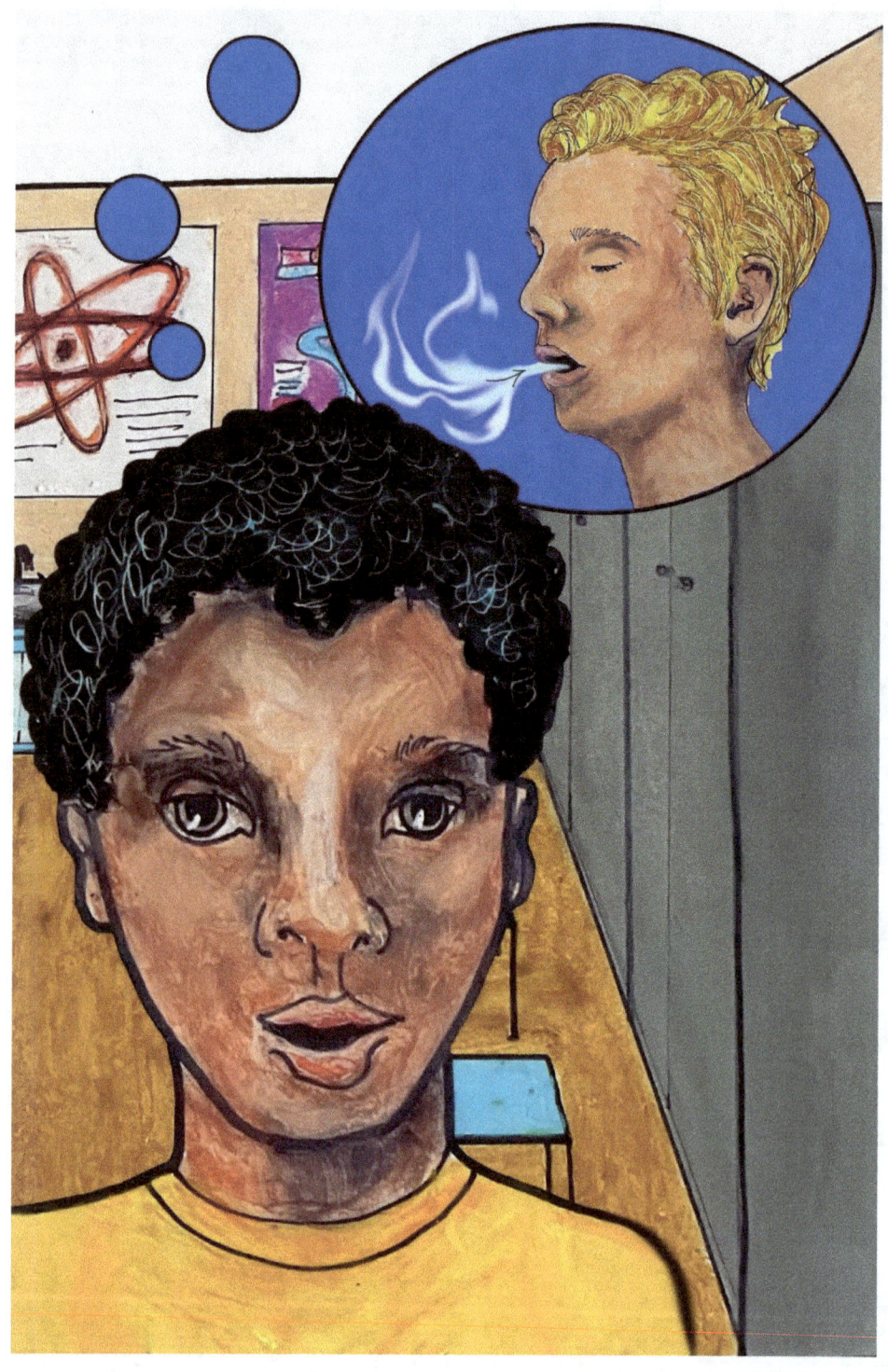

Ekon raises his hand, and Nurse Dorothea calls on him to talk. "In the past, I noticed that when I would get angry, my heart rate would increase a lot. I learned to do deep breathing and get relaxed, which slows my heart rate down. I now use anger as a sign to tell me that I need to start deep breathing. It has helped me a lot."

"Deep breathing is a skill we should all probably learn," says Nurse Dorothea.

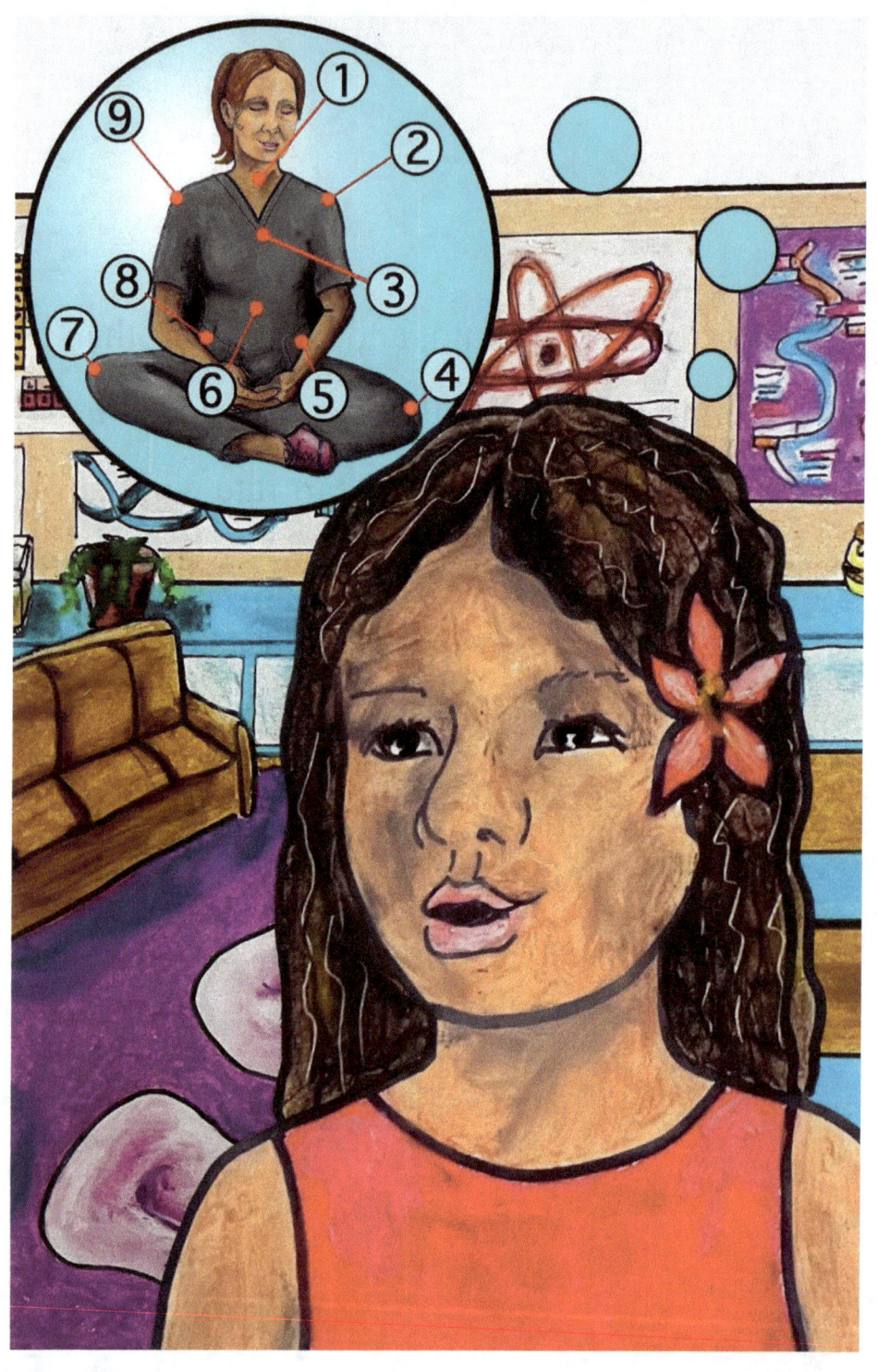

Kalani raises her hand, and Nurse Dorothea calls on her to talk. "I've found that progressive muscle relaxation helps me relax when I get angry. I do this by tensing muscles one at a time around my body and then relax them. After I do the whole body, it really helps."

"Thanks for sharing," says Nurse Dorothea.

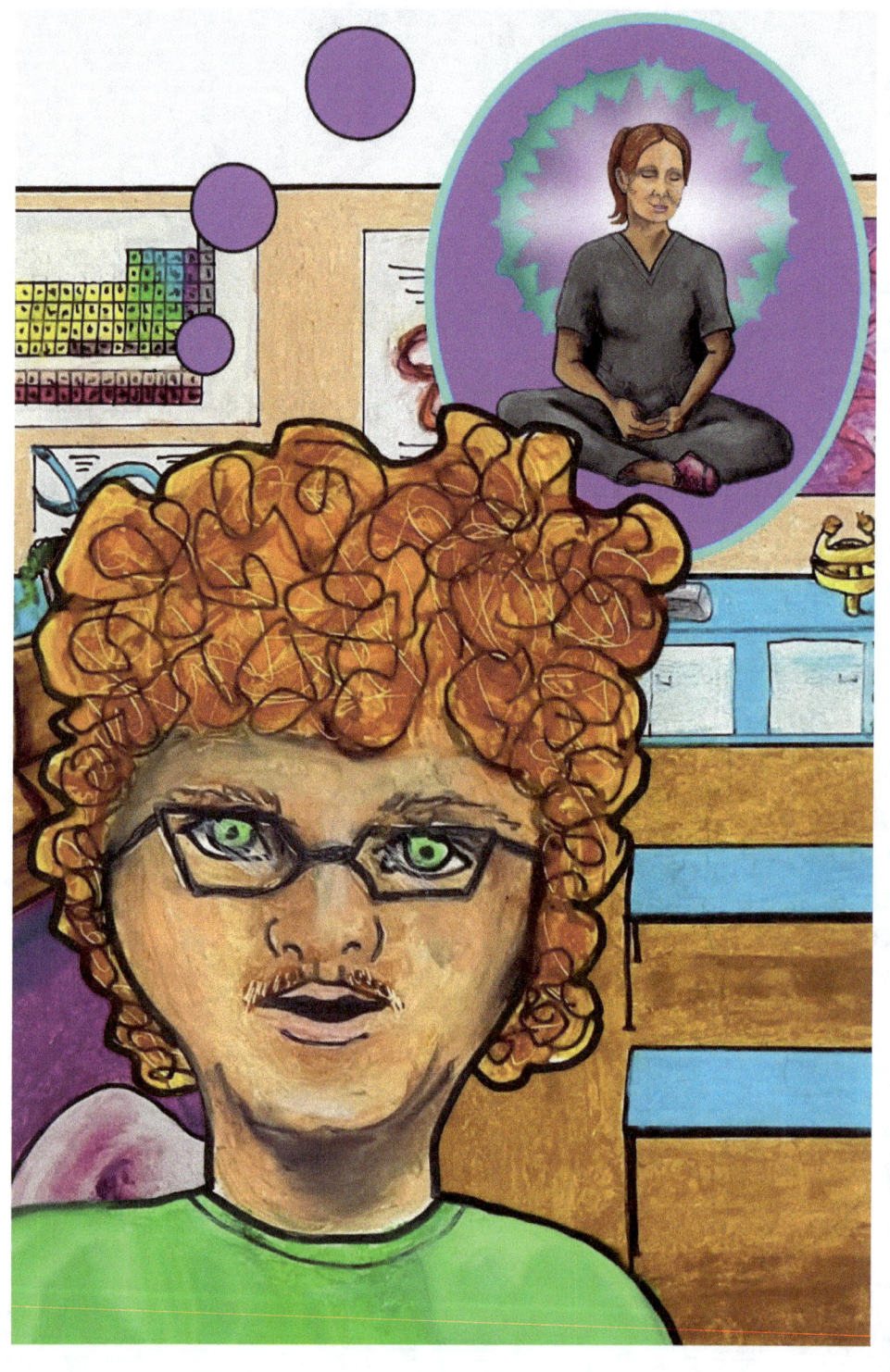

Connor raises his hand, and Nurse Dorothea calls on him to talk. "When I get angry, I use it as a sign for me to go by myself somewhere and meditate. I like to say certain mantras repeatedly such as, 'I am strong enough,' 'I am capable and will find the right solution,' and 'I can face my fears and anxiety and find peace.' "

"Meditation can help a lot of people, and we should all try it sometime," says Nurse Dorothea.

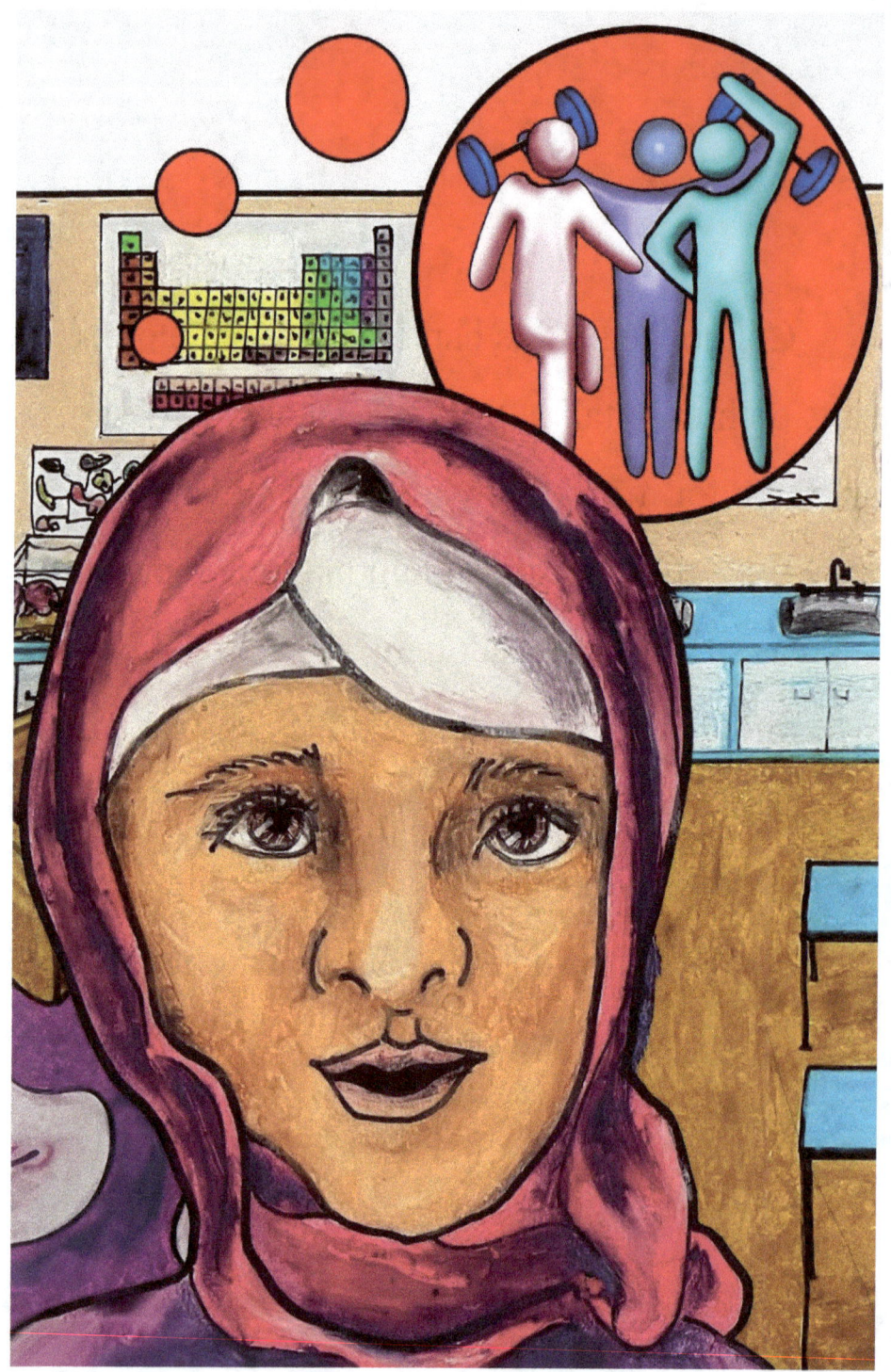

Fatima raises her hand, and Nurse Dorothea calls on her to talk. "When I get angry, I start exercising such as doing push-ups and sit-ups. I have some barbells at home which I also use sometimes. They are 10 pounds each, and I can do about 20 curls in each arm. Exercising lets me take out my angry energy in a useful way."

"Science shows that exercising regularly each week can help with good health. We should all try to find some exercises that we enjoy and then do them often. They should be exercises that increase our heart rate and make us sweat. Even fast walking can be good exercise. Swimming is very helpful for people who need to worry about too much stress on their joints, like their knees because they may be obese," says Nurse Dorothea.

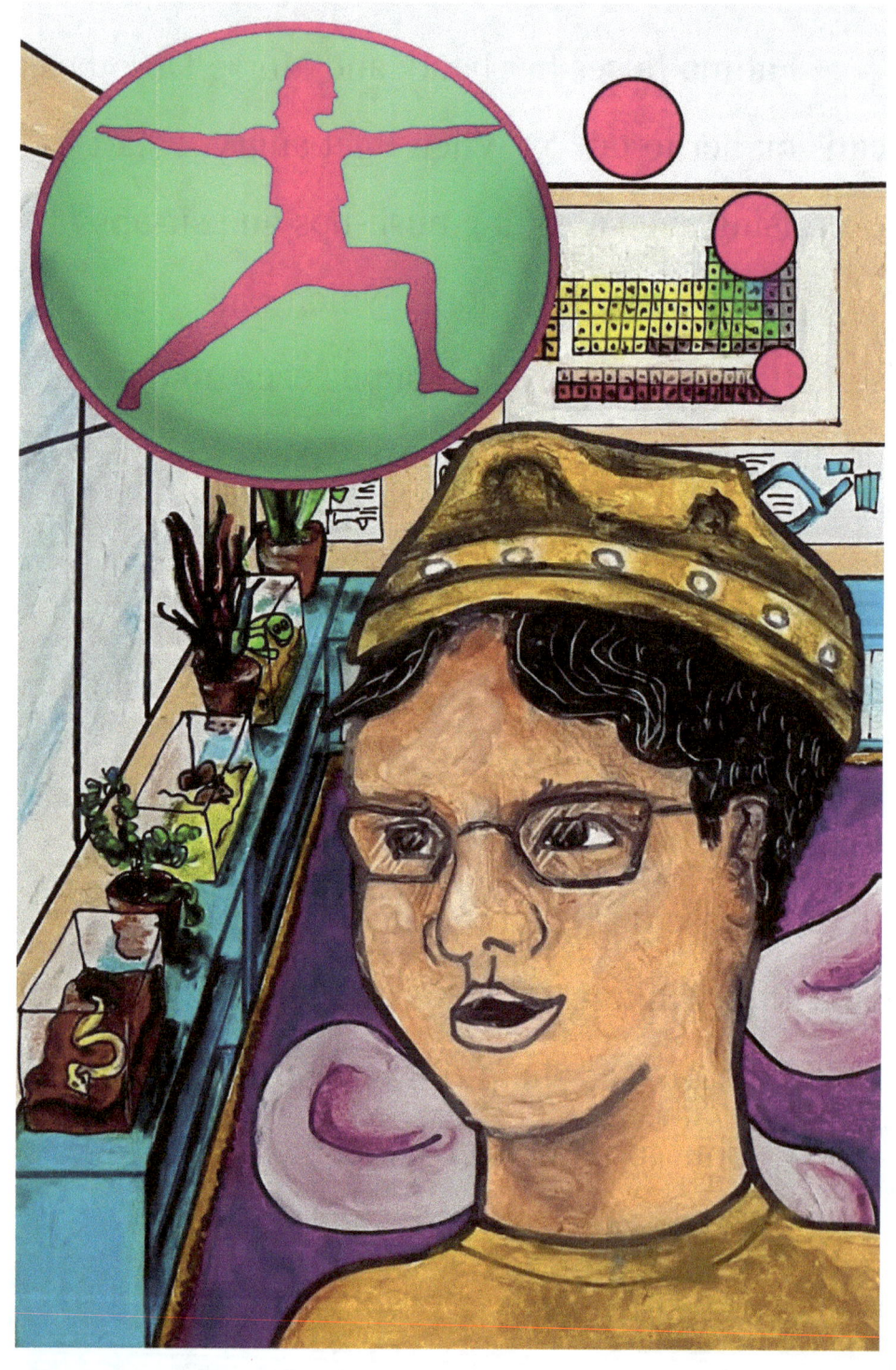

Azamat raises his hand, and Nurse Dorothea calls on him to talk. "My mom introduced me to yoga, which is basically controlled slow movements of the body into different positions, which also helps with stretching. I've done yoga sometimes when I was angry, and it helped me relax."

"Yoga is very enjoyable for some people and worth doing a couple of times to see if it's right for you. Just because you may not like the coping skill after doing it once doesn't mean that it's not good for you. Sometimes, we have to do a coping skill several times to see if we find it enjoyable," says Nurse Dorothea.

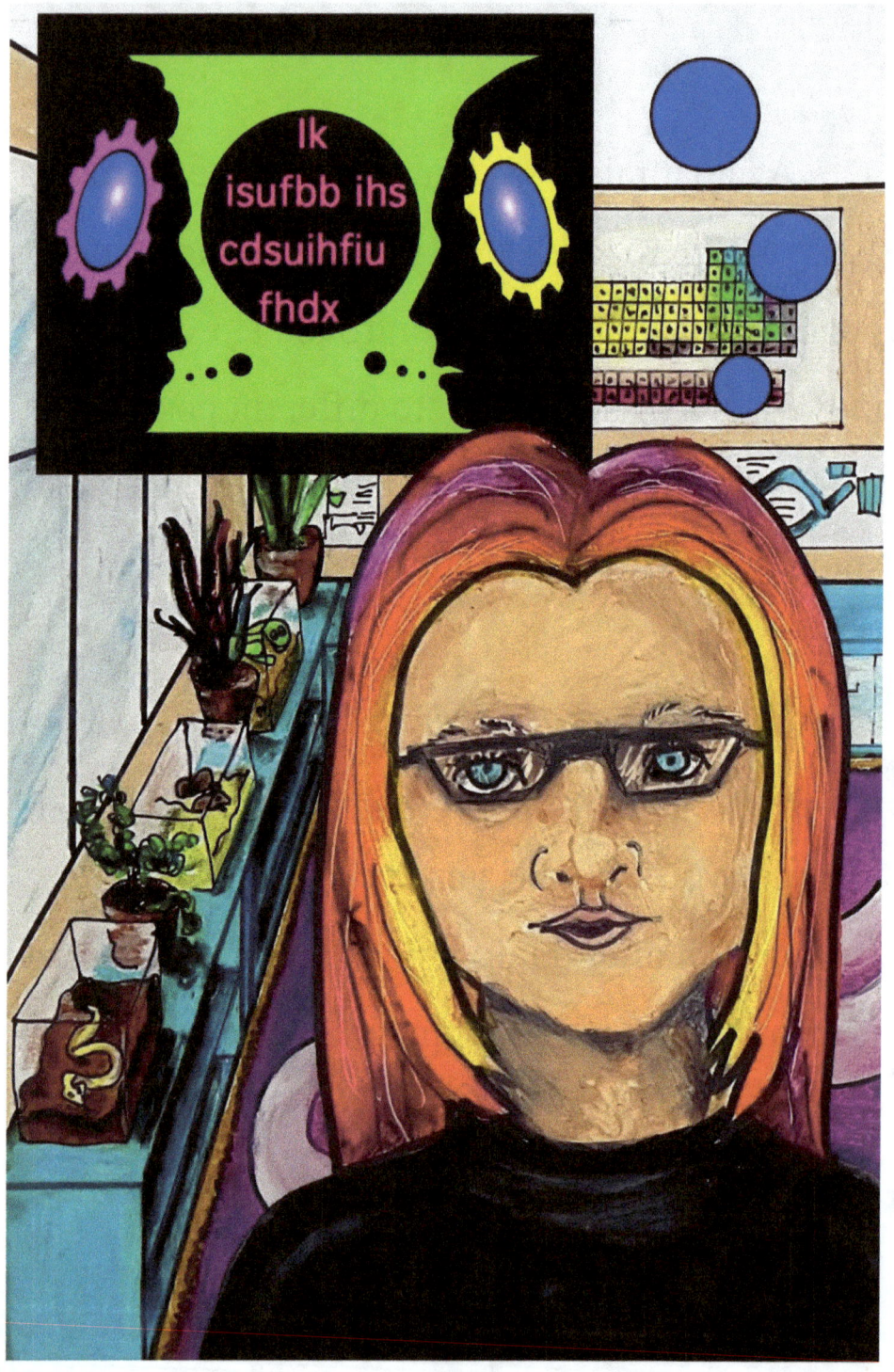

Juniper raises her hand, and Nurse Dorothea calls on her to talk. "I've found that talking to someone about what is making me angry helps me to calm down. It's nice to have someone who I can talk to and just let me vent. Just having someone listen is really nice."

"Having someone to vent to is important. You must be careful and do extra things for those people to show you appreciate them, since venting all the time to the same person could wear them out, and they may avoid you," says Nurse Dorothea.

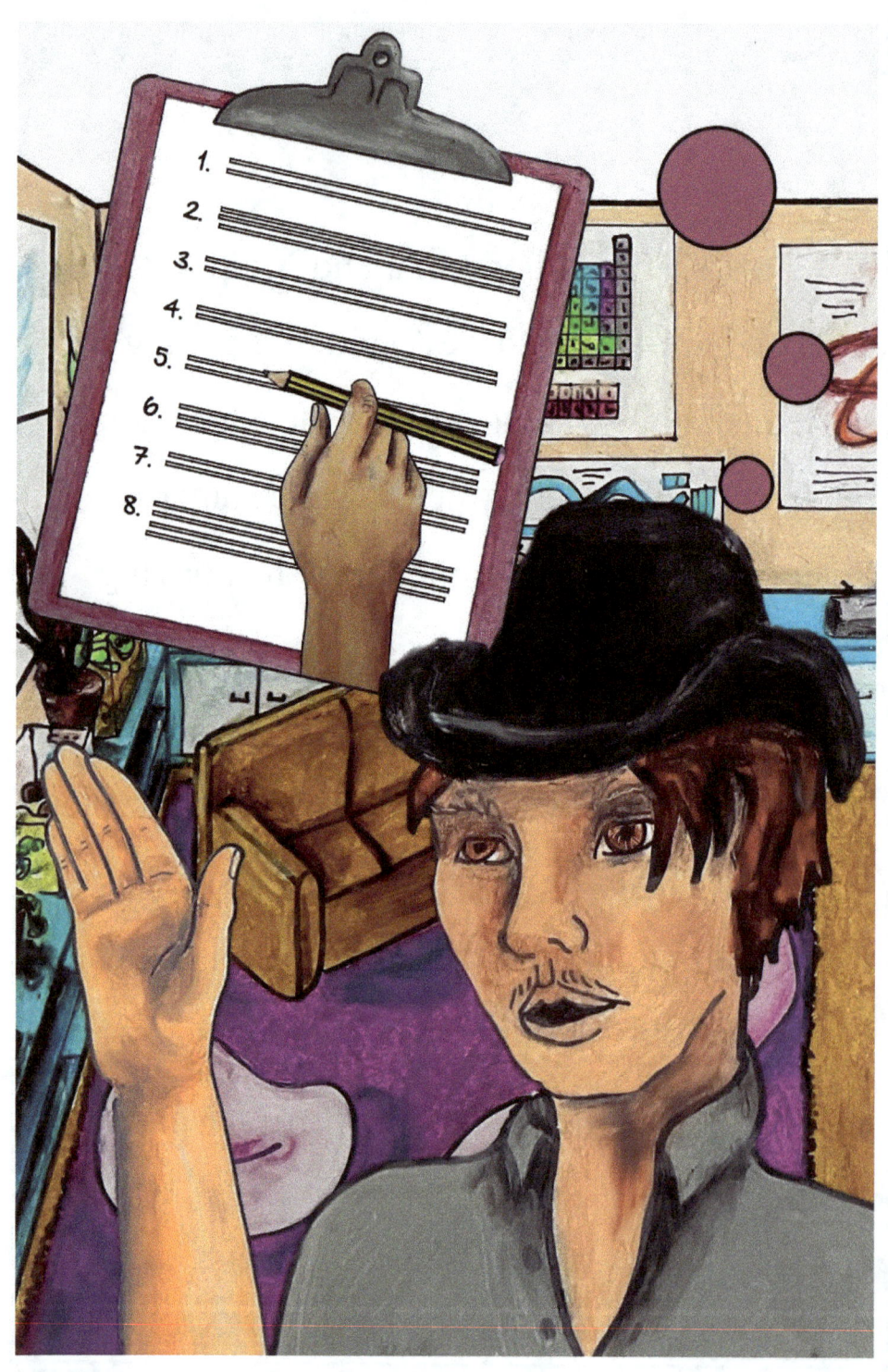

Wyatt raises his hand, and Nurse Dorothea calls on him to talk. "When I get angry, it has helped me to write down goals to help resolve whatever was making me angry. Having goals to accomplish things helps me feel I'm making progress on my mental health journey."

"Giving yourself goal-focused therapy is a great idea!" says Nurse Dorothea.

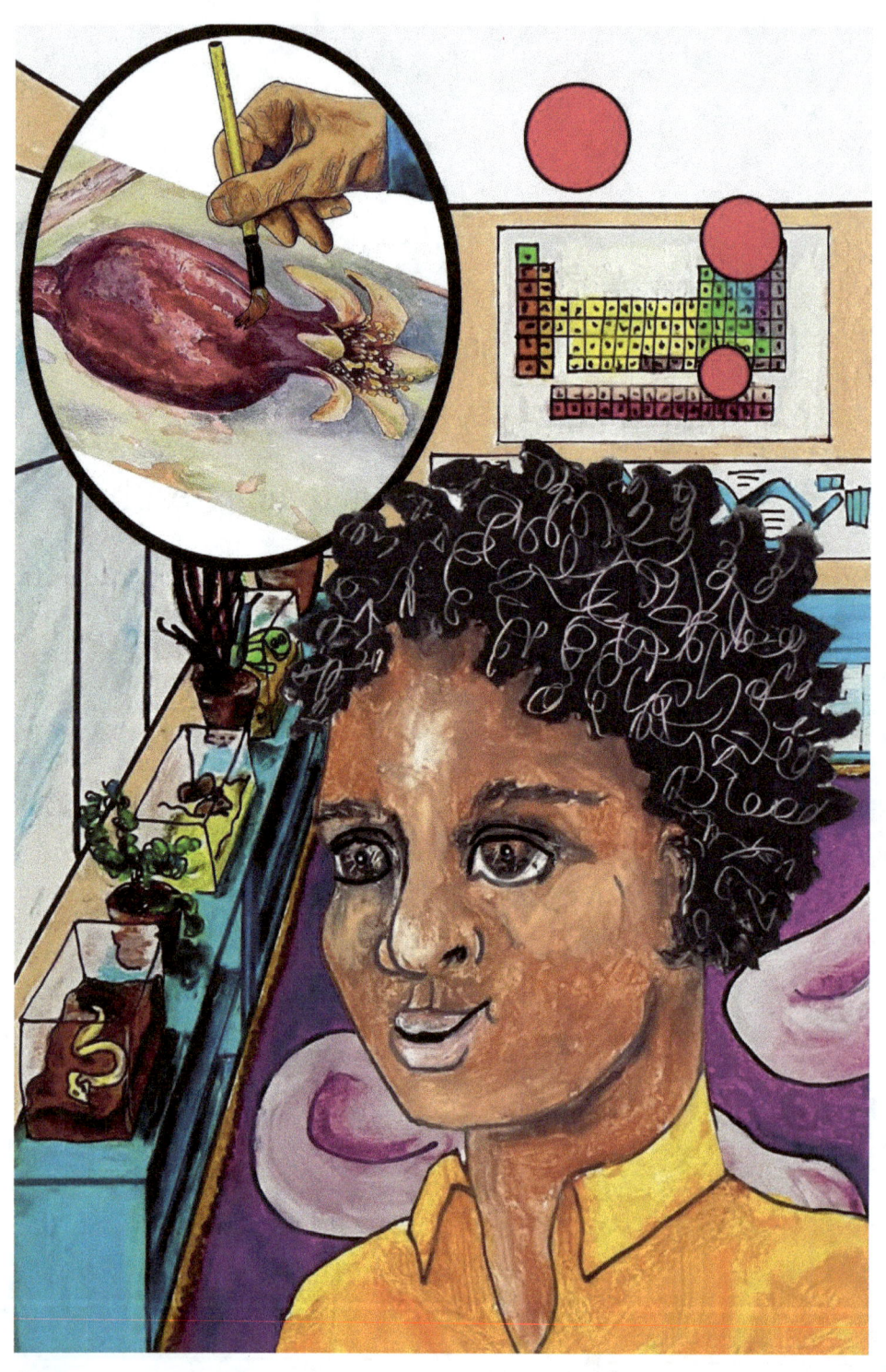

Amari raises his hand, and Nurse Dorothea calls on him to talk. "I like to use my anger energy to draw or paint. I seem to be able to convert my anger energy into creative energy and have made some really beautiful things by doing that. It makes me feel better after I create something beautiful."

"Transforming anger into creativity is wonderful," says Nurse Dorothea.

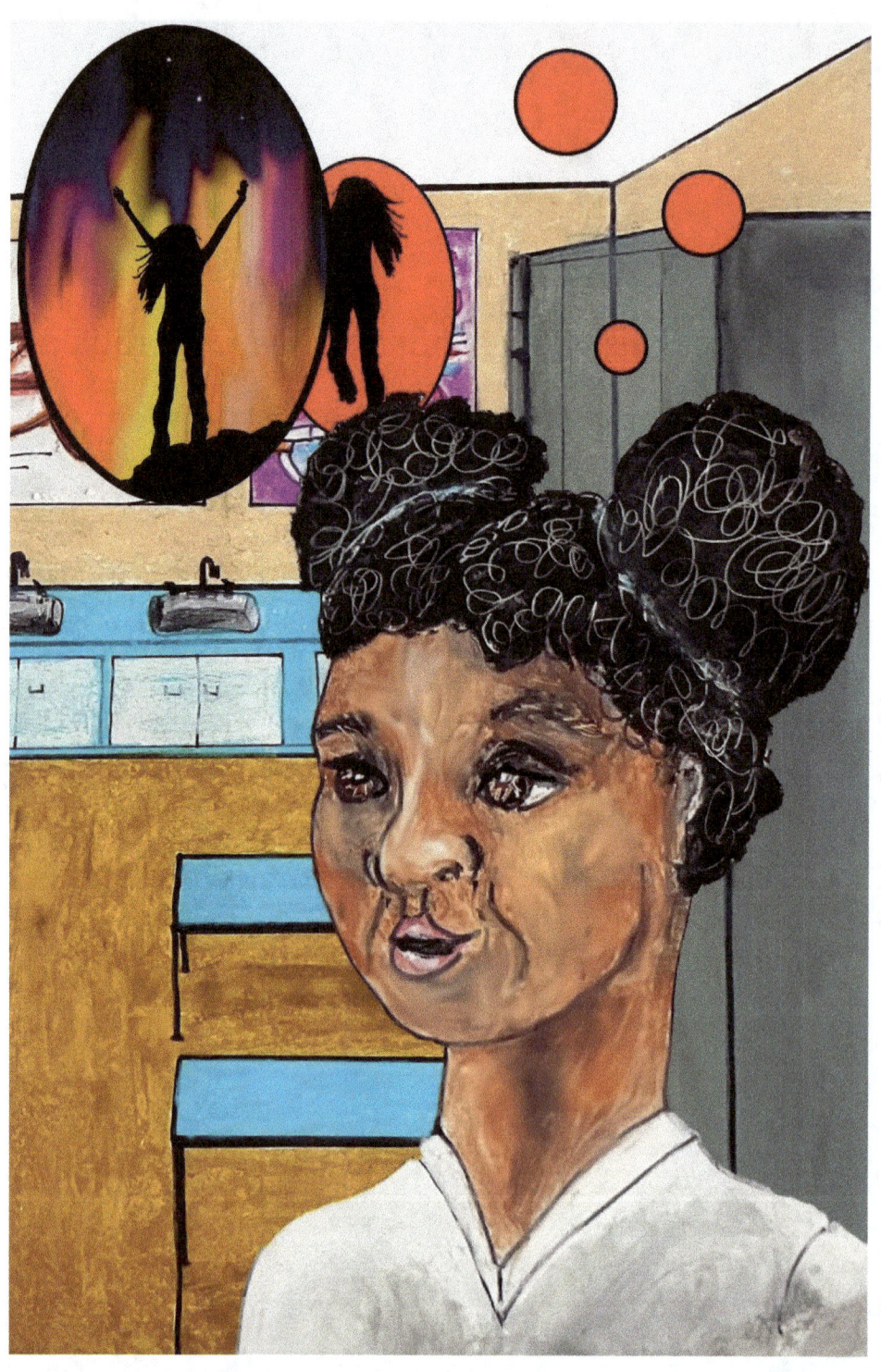

Amisha raises her hand, and Nurse Dorothea calls on her to talk. "I've found that what helps me when I'm angry is to step away and get a change of scenery. Just being away from the situation or environment that led me into anger helps me stop being angry and calm down."

"Sometimes changing one's environment can be the main thing that will help someone relax," says Nurse Dorothea.

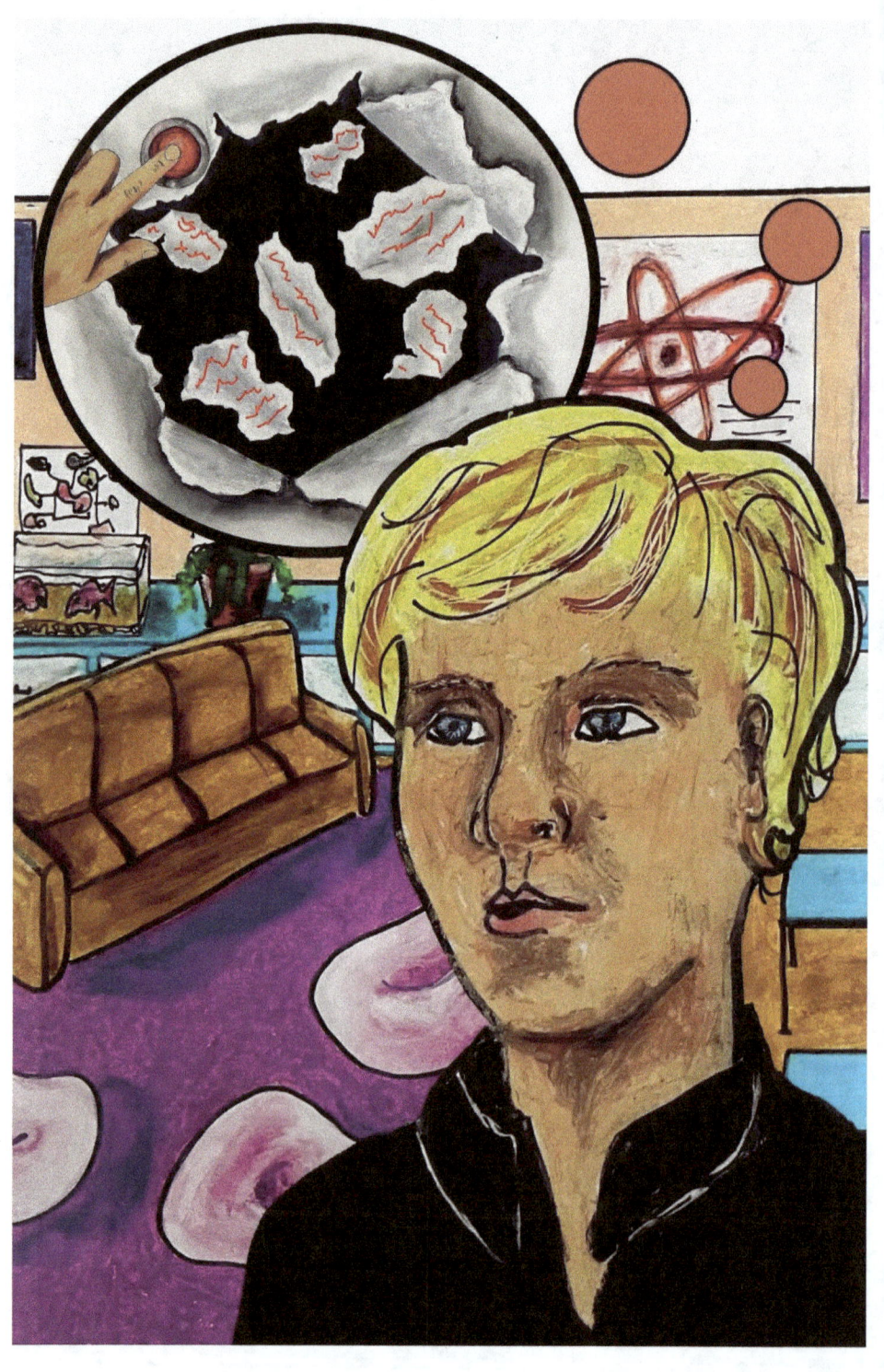

Dimitry raises his hand, and Nurse Dorothea calls on him to talk. "Something I've done in the past is to write down my triggers for anger and then rip up the piece of paper. It's like I'm destroying my triggers, and it makes me feel a little better. It doesn't make it go away completely, but it helps."

"Sometimes every little bit helps, and taking our anger down a notch is enough for us to better manage that emotion," says Nurse Dorothea.

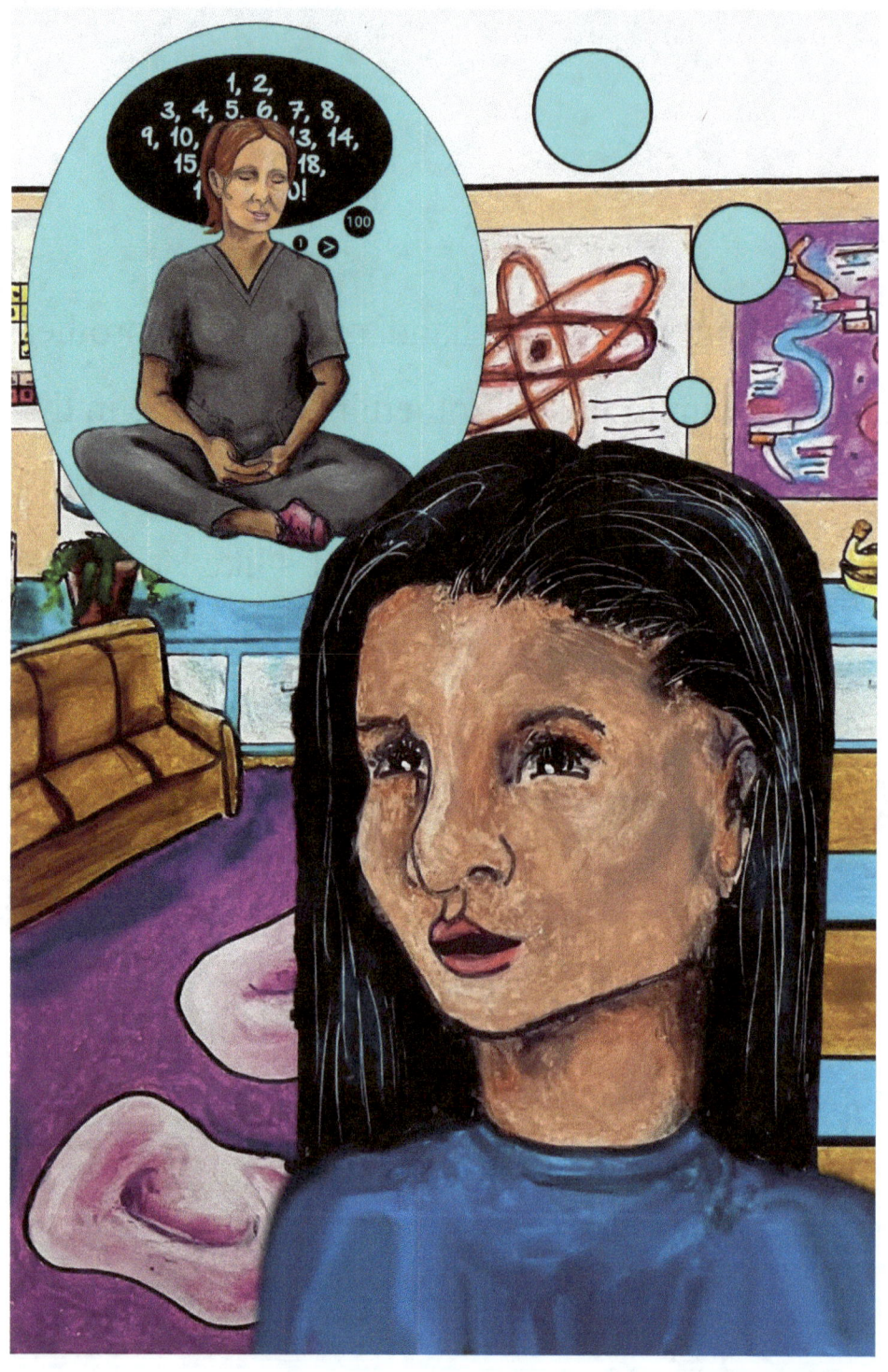

Diwa raises her hand, and Nurse Dorothea calls on her to talk. "Once when I was angry, I counted down from 100 to zero. It helped distract me and helped me regain my peace."

"Counting down can be an effective coping skill sometimes for some people," says Nurse Dorothea.

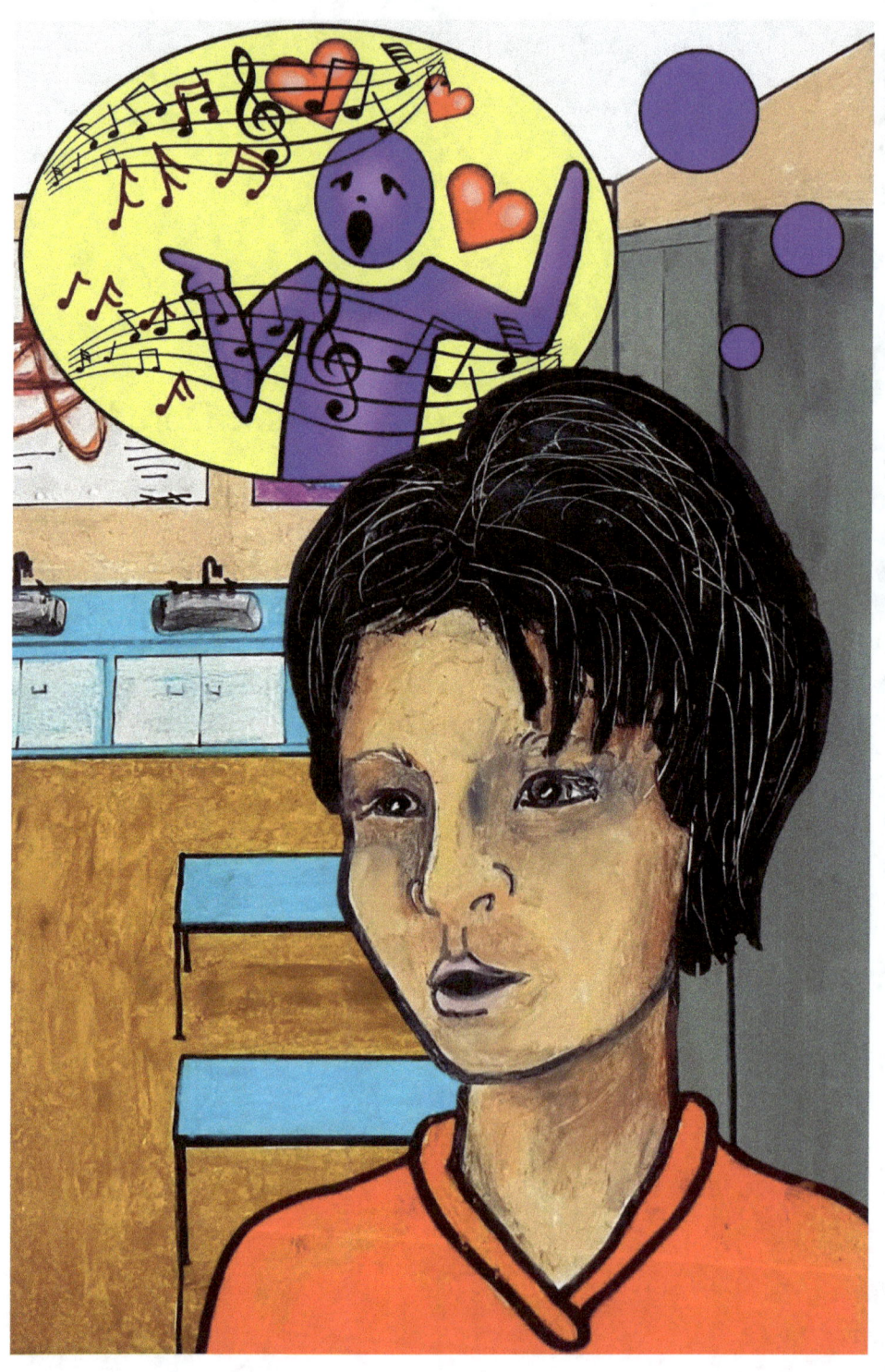

Kenji raises his hand, and Nurse Dorothea calls on him to talk. "I've done something interesting with music relaxation. When I get angry, I'll listen to angry music for a little bit, then I'll change it up to be more relaxing music. I think the angry music helps my mind get in tune with something, and then switching to relaxing music helps me transition out of anger."

"That is interesting. Maybe you could be a scientist one day and create an experiment to see if that technique is effective with everyone," says Nurse Dorothea.

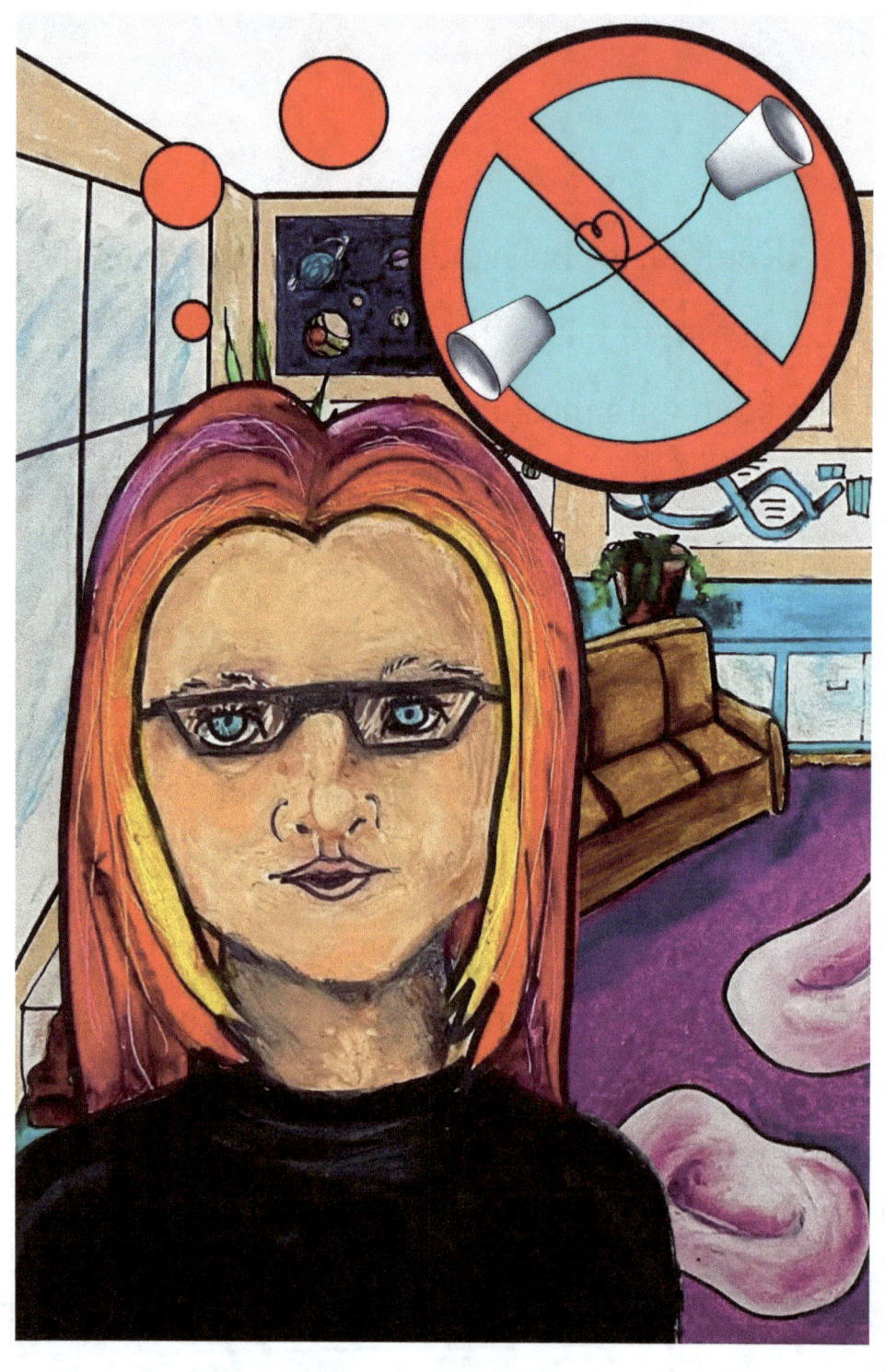

Juniper raises her hand, and Nurse Dorothea calls on her to talk. "When I get angry, I've learned to just be quiet because I'm pretty sure I'm going to say something that I'll regret. And if I regret something I've said, I may get angry with myself, so the anger just continues. Silence has really helped."

"That is good self-control to stop talking. Great work!" says Nurse Dorothea.

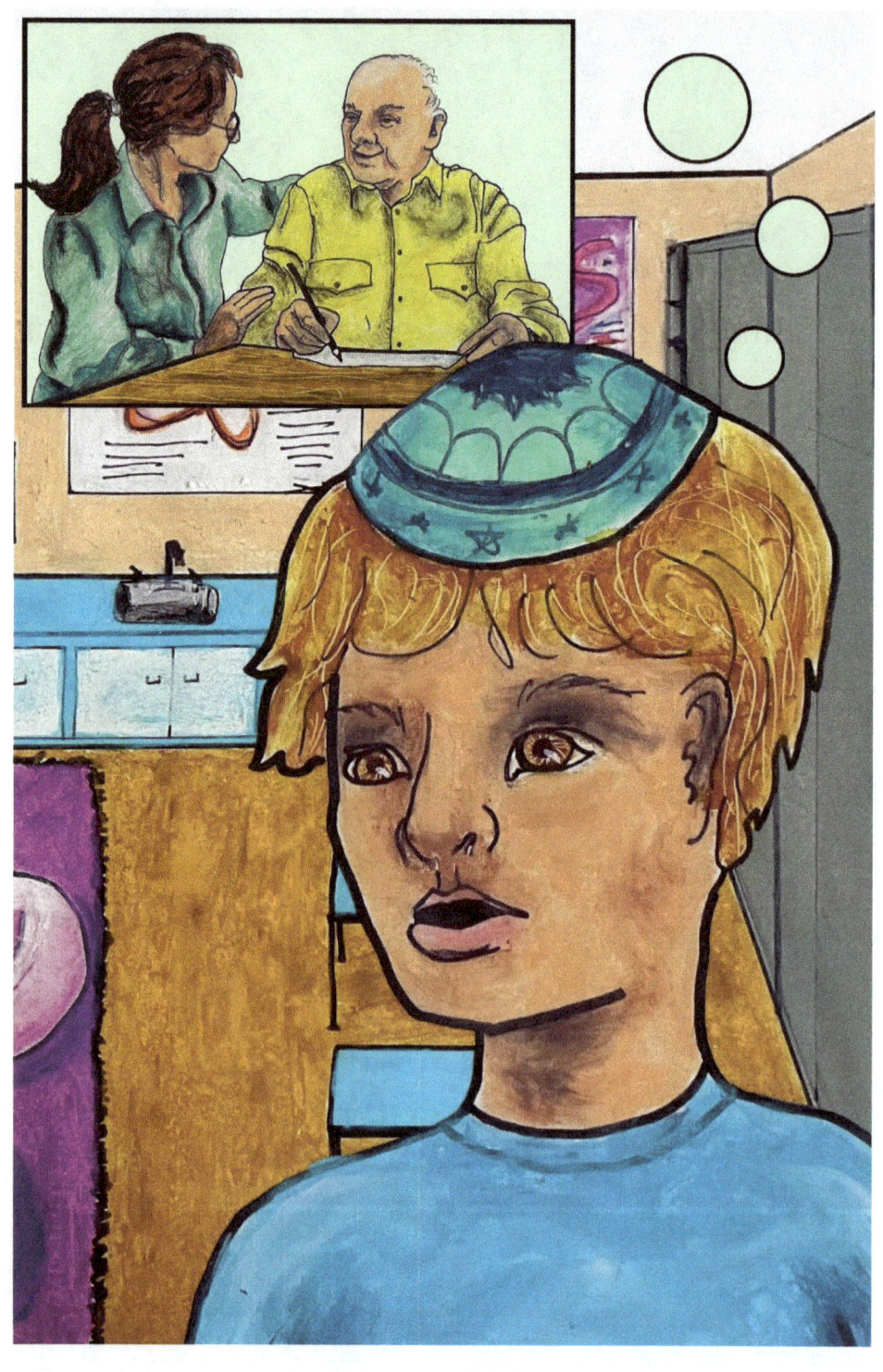

Levi raises his hand, and Nurse Dorothea calls on him to talk. "I've gotten angry in the past, and I chose to do something nice for someone to help me have a more pleasant feeling. It really felt nice to help someone, and the other person felt nice that something good was being done for them. That good feeling helped wash away my anger."

"A change in emotions can be effective in managing anger," says Nurse Dorothea.

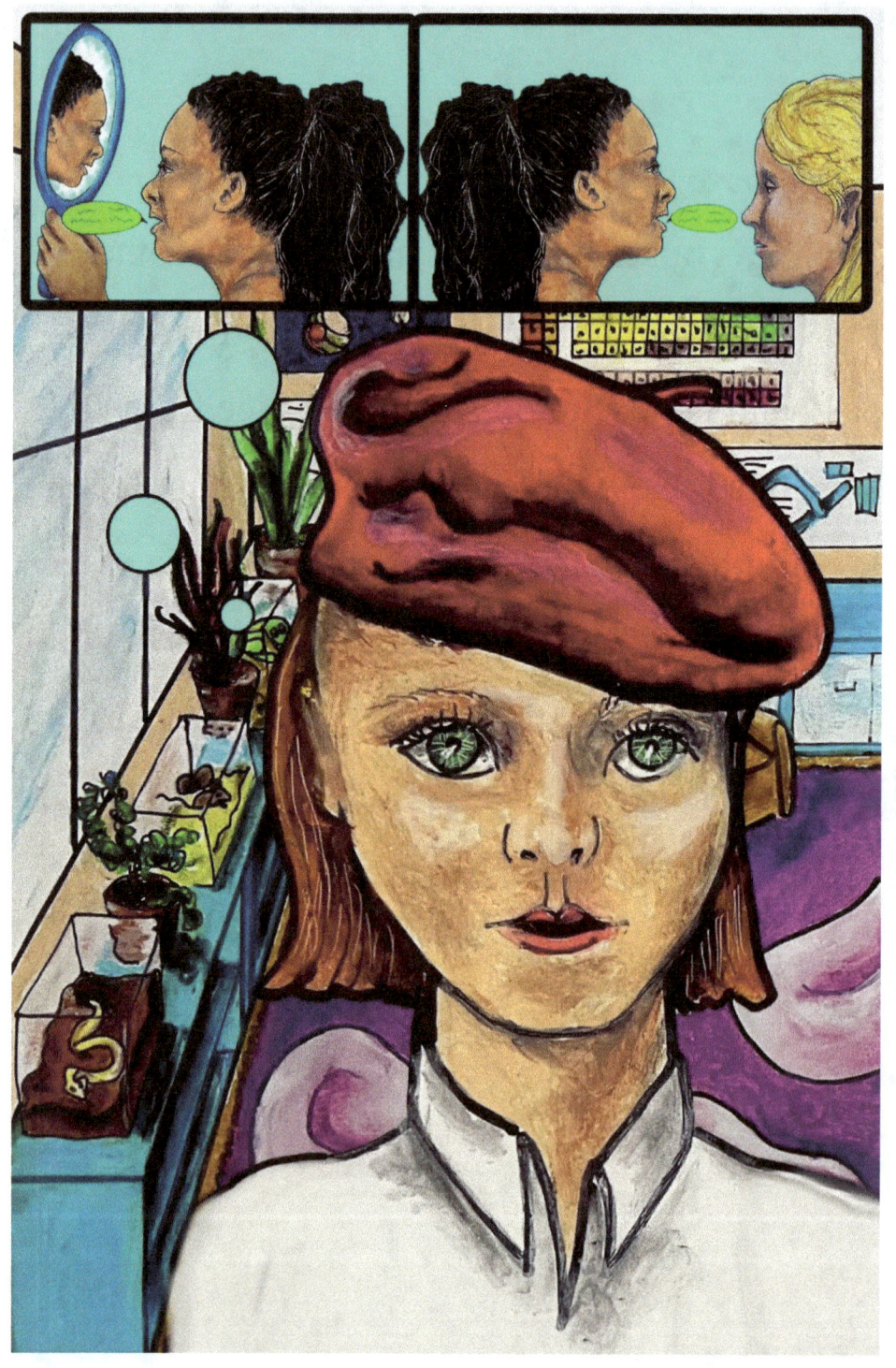

Marie raises her hand, and Nurse Dorothea calls on her to talk. "Once, I was very angry and wanted to tell someone how I felt. I asked a friend to rehearse the conversation with me. I tried to talk calmly to my friend as if they were the other person, and then my friend talked back to me to try to imitate what the other person might say. When I approached the other person and talked to them about my feelings, I had more control of my anger and didn't raise my voice. I stayed calm and was able to effectively communicate my feelings which helped resolve the situation."

"That's a great idea. Rehearsing a situation that may get you angry so that you can manage your emotions is a key to anger management," says Nurse Dorothea.

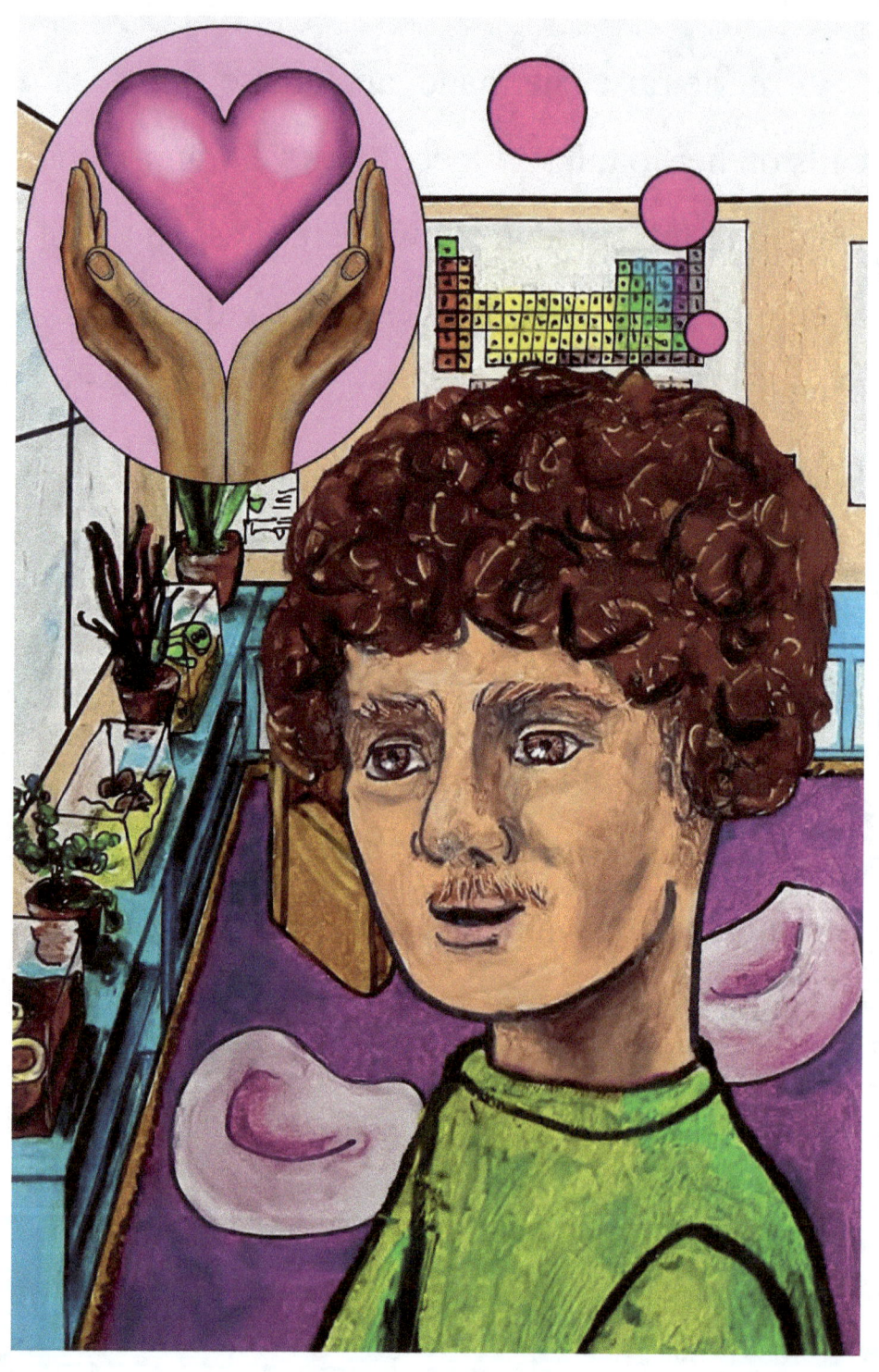

Gustavo raises his hand, and Nurse Dorothea calls on him to talk. "In the past, when I was angry, I tried to refocus my attention away from my feelings and triggers toward things I was grateful for in my life. Changing my thoughts helped me regain control."

"Gratitude is a powerful emotion, and sometimes it must be a deliberate thought and feeling. Saying you're thankful for something when you don't have the feeling doesn't mean you're not being true to yourself. You are just using a tool, which is gratitude, to generate a different feeling so that you can move forward in your journey," says Nurse Dorothea.

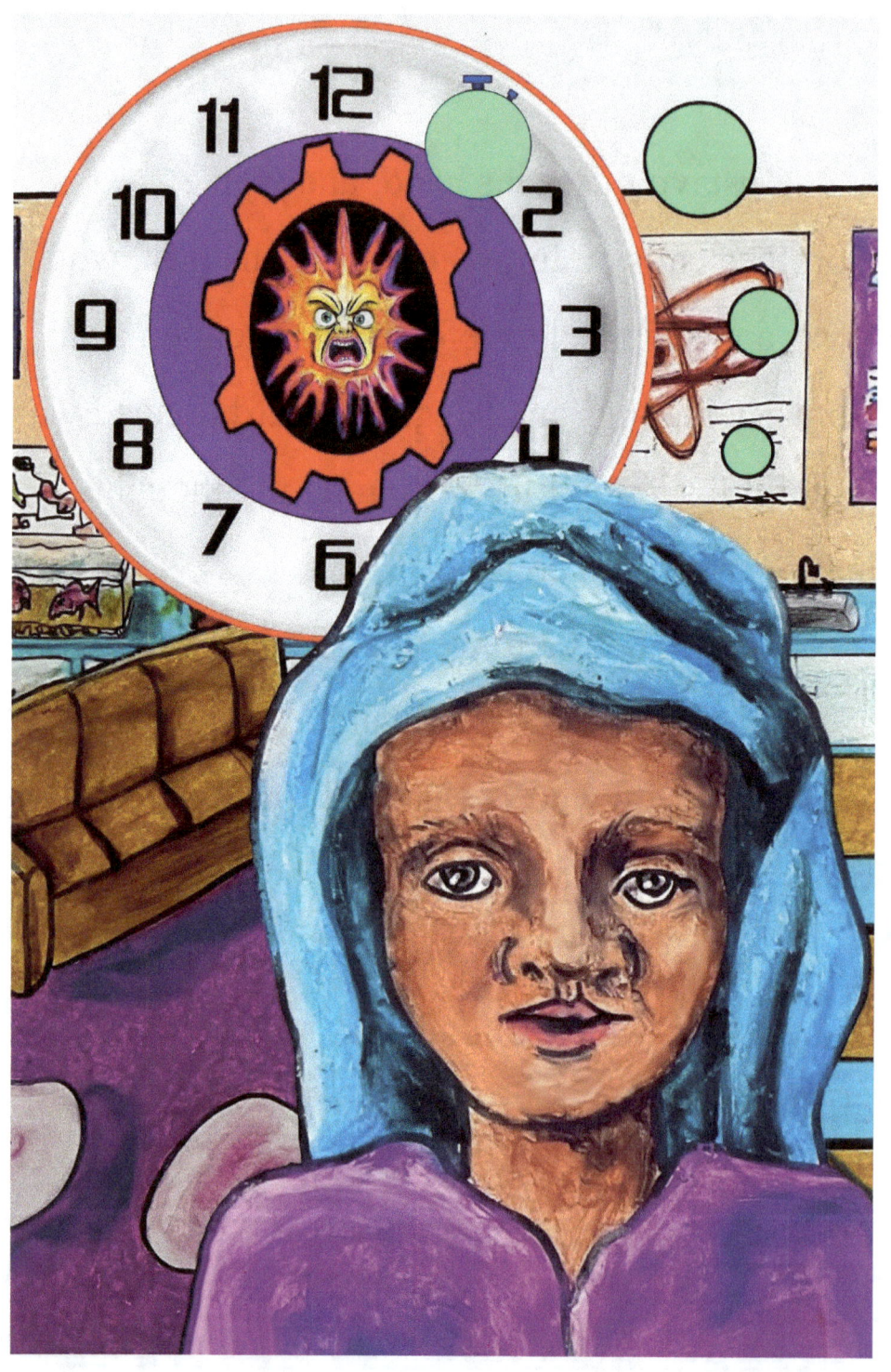

Yuliana raises her hand, and Nurse Dorothea calls on her to talk. "What has worked for me in the past, which I learned from my dad is to set a timer and choose to be angry for only the amount of time that is set. After the timer goes off, I tell myself it's time to change emotions, and it has worked."

"Allowing yourself to feel angry is important since it is a natural emotion, so it is great you have learned that skill," says Nurse Dorothea.

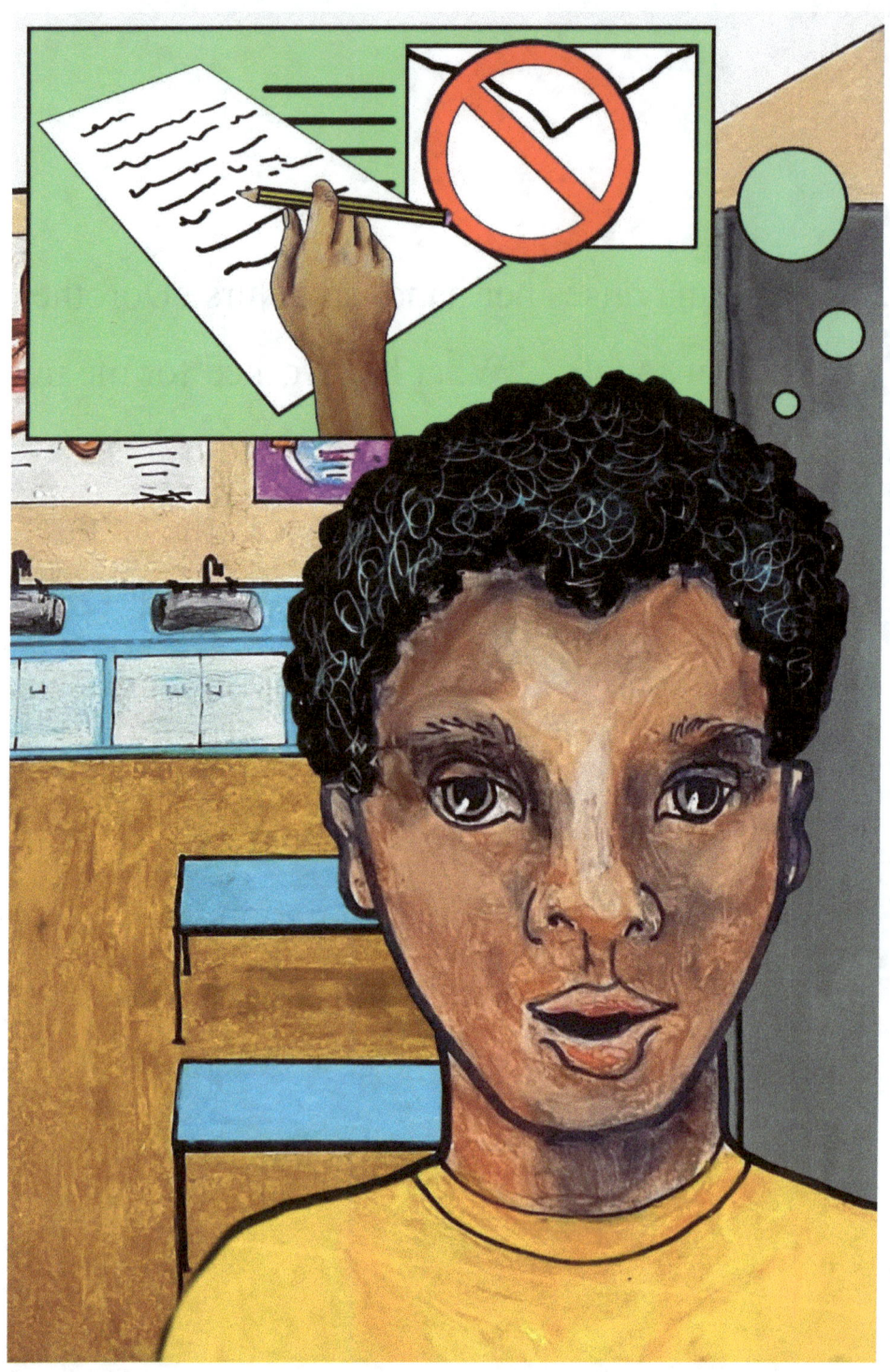

Dimitry raises his hand, and Nurse Dorothea calls on him to talk. "Once, I was really angry at someone, and I wrote a letter to them. I said a lot of mean things in the letter, but I didn't give it to them. It helped me get my thoughts out of my head."

"Journaling can be very therapeutic. Some people may want to rip it up and throw it away so that others do not read, since it contains a lot of raw emotions, and you may not really mean it," says Nurse Dorothea.

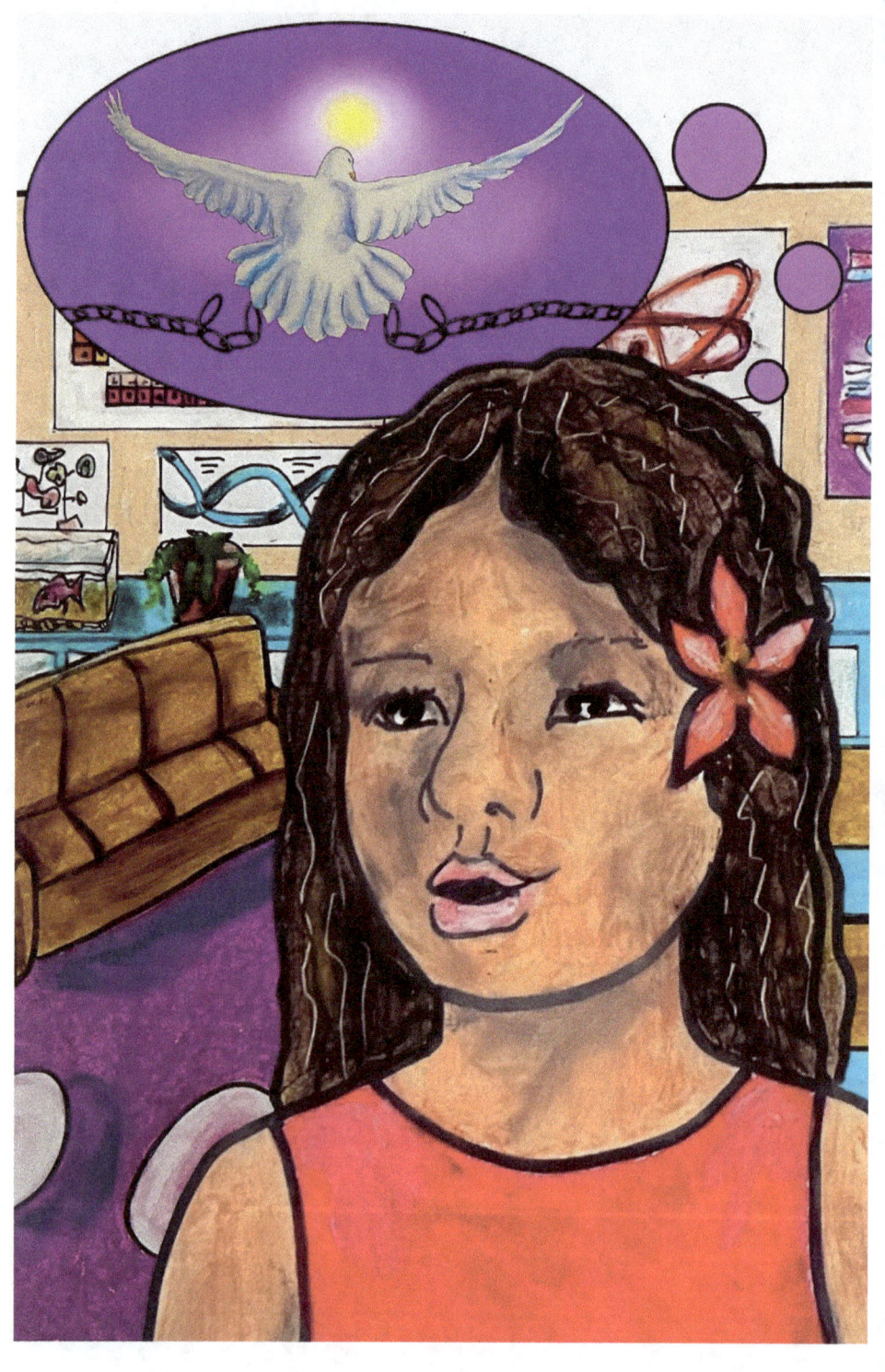

Kalani raises her hand, and Nurse Dorothea calls on her to talk. "My religion teaches me to practice forgiveness. I think forgiveness is a skill that must be exercised to be good at it. It's hard sometimes, but forgiving can release you from your anger."

"You're right that forgiveness is a skill. Not many people are great at it once they start, but the more you do it, the better you will be," says Nurse Dorothea.

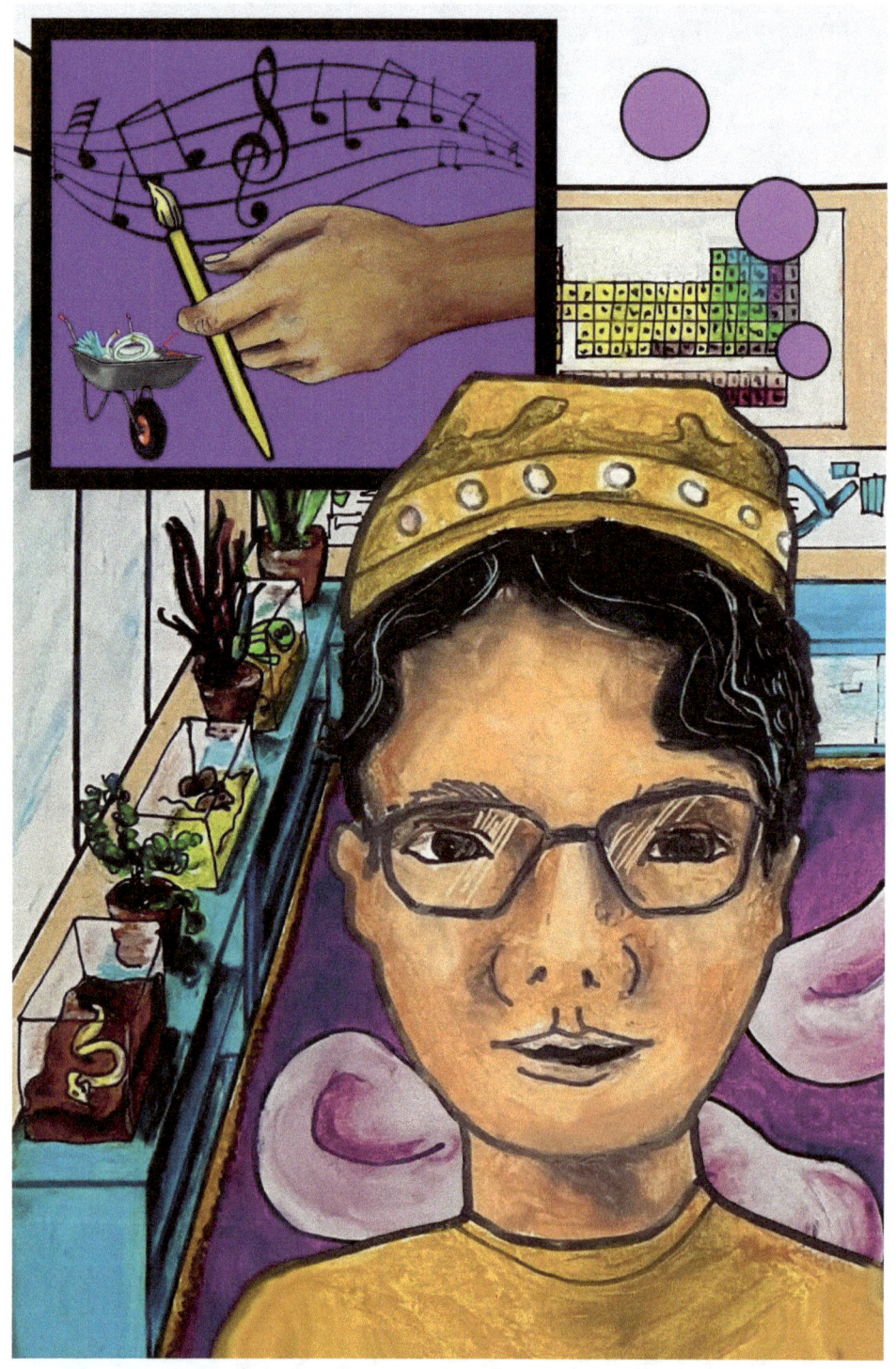

Azamat raises his hand, and Nurse Dorothea calls on him to talk. "I do creative things with my anger, like play music, paint, and garden."

"Using our anger as a creative force can be helpful for not just ourselves, but also for society, since our creative products can help other people," says Nurse Dorothea.

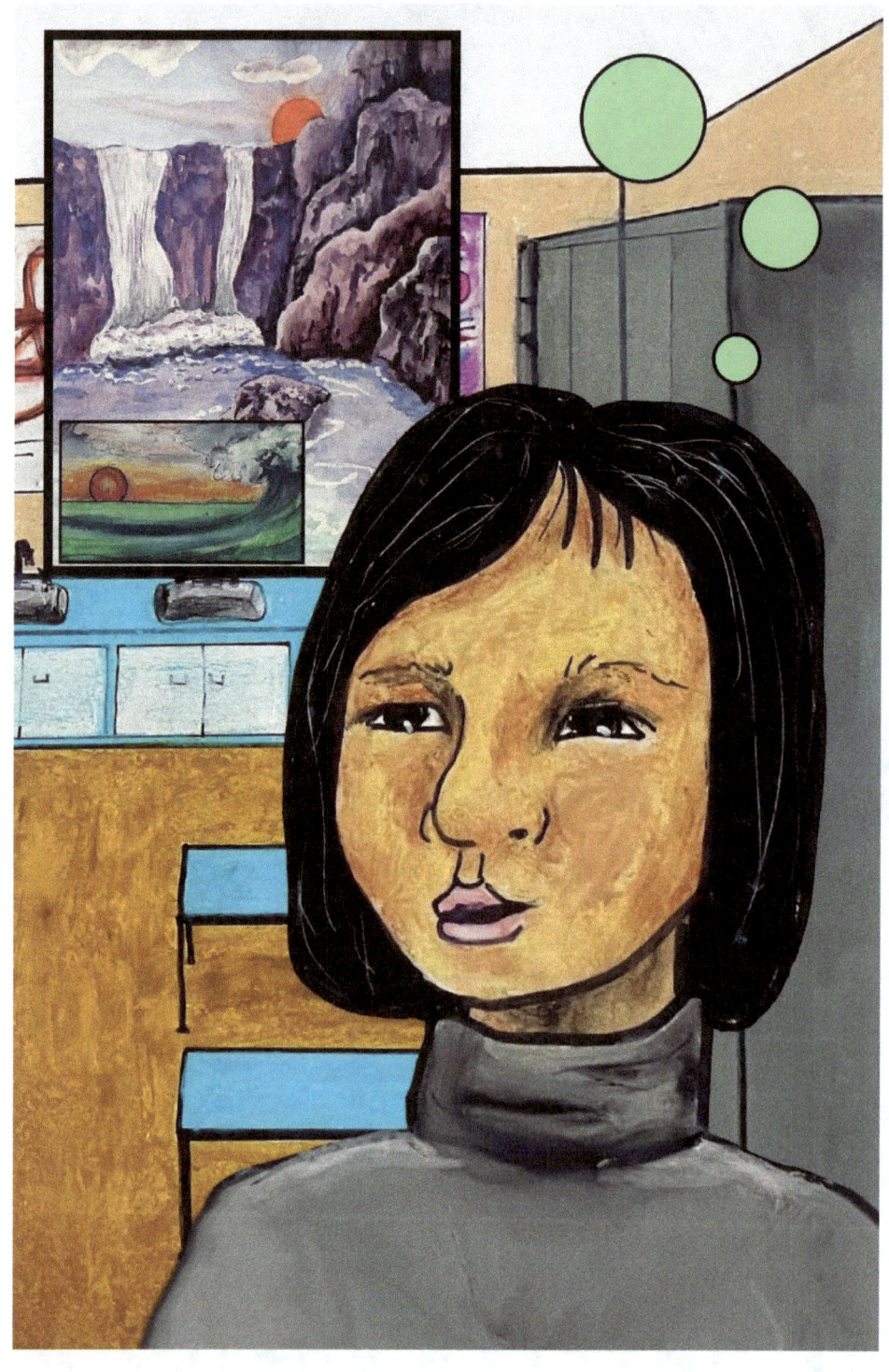

Lian raises her hand, and Nurse Dorothea calls on her to talk. "I like to go on hikes and enjoy nature when I get angry or frustrated with things. Nature is relaxing to me, and I love it."

"Mother Nature has created some amazing scenery and things to enjoy. Let's be appreciative for the world around us, and use it to regain our mental equilibrium," says Nurse Dorothea.

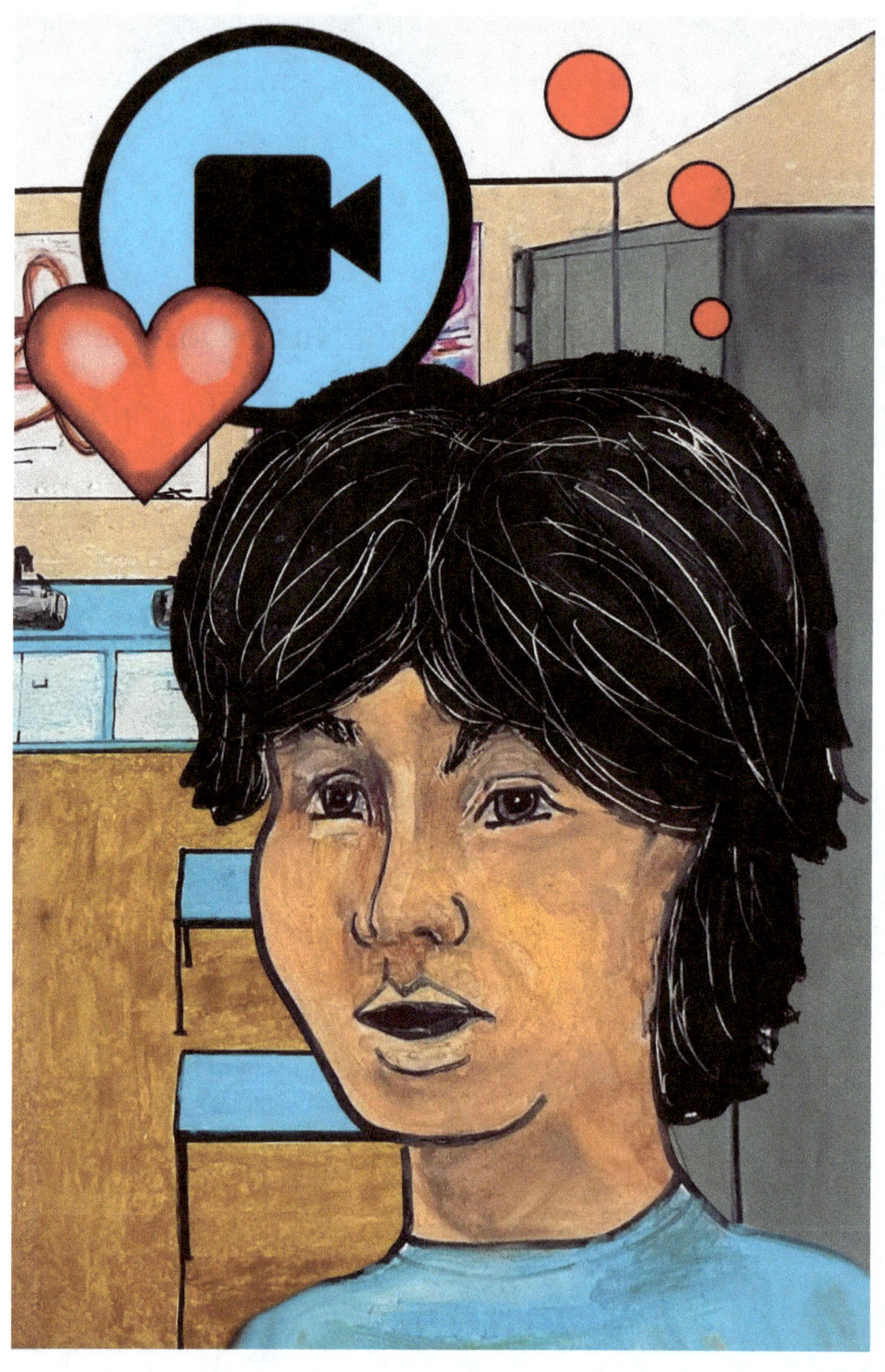

Ji Ho raises his hand, and Nurse Dorothea calls on him to talk. "Something that has helped me is to watch my favorite movie when I get angry. I must have seen it 100 times, and it helps me change my mood."

"Watching or listening to something comforting can be very helpful," says Nurse Dorothea.

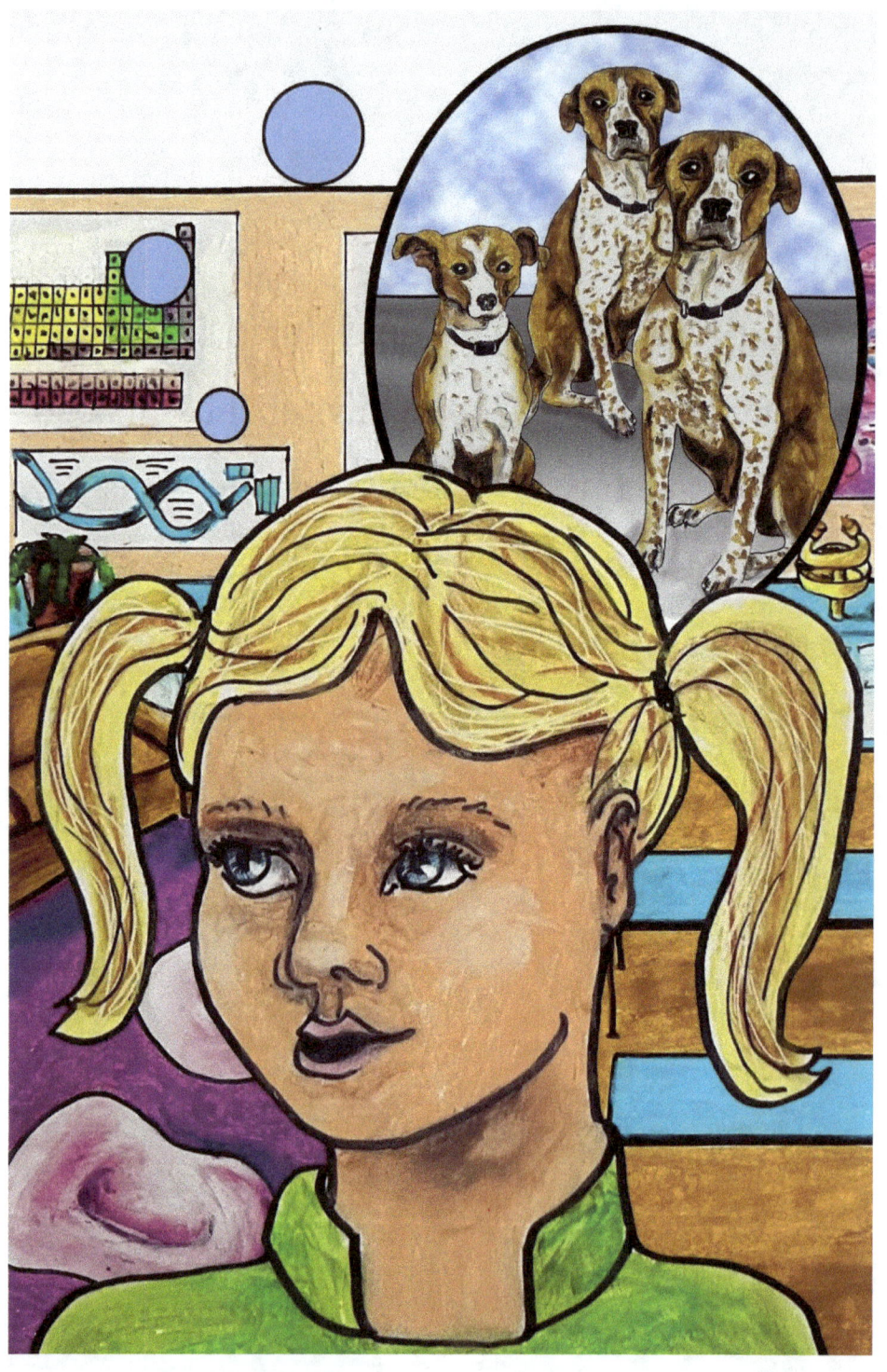

Frida raises her hand, and Nurse Dorothea calls on her to talk. "When I get frustrated, I like to spend more time with my pets. They are very loving and let me pet them as much as I want, which helps me to relax."

"Pets are an important part of human life, and we should care for them properly," says Nurse Dorothea.

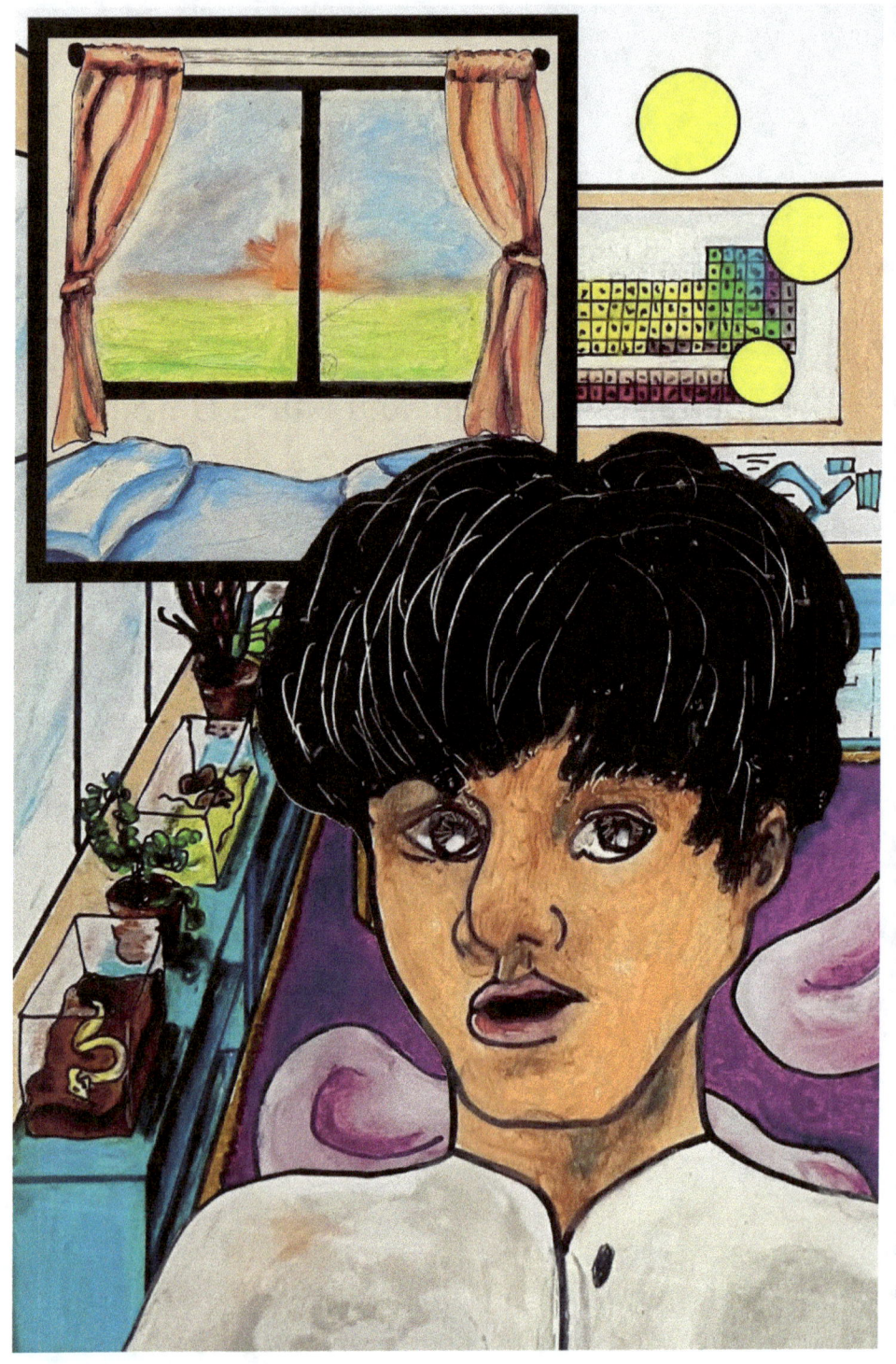

Antonio raises his hand, and Nurse Dorothea calls on him to talk. "When I get really frustrated at home, I like to take a short nap. It helps me to stop thinking about my triggers and gets me back to a restful place."

"Rest is important for the mind and the body," says Nurse Dorothea.

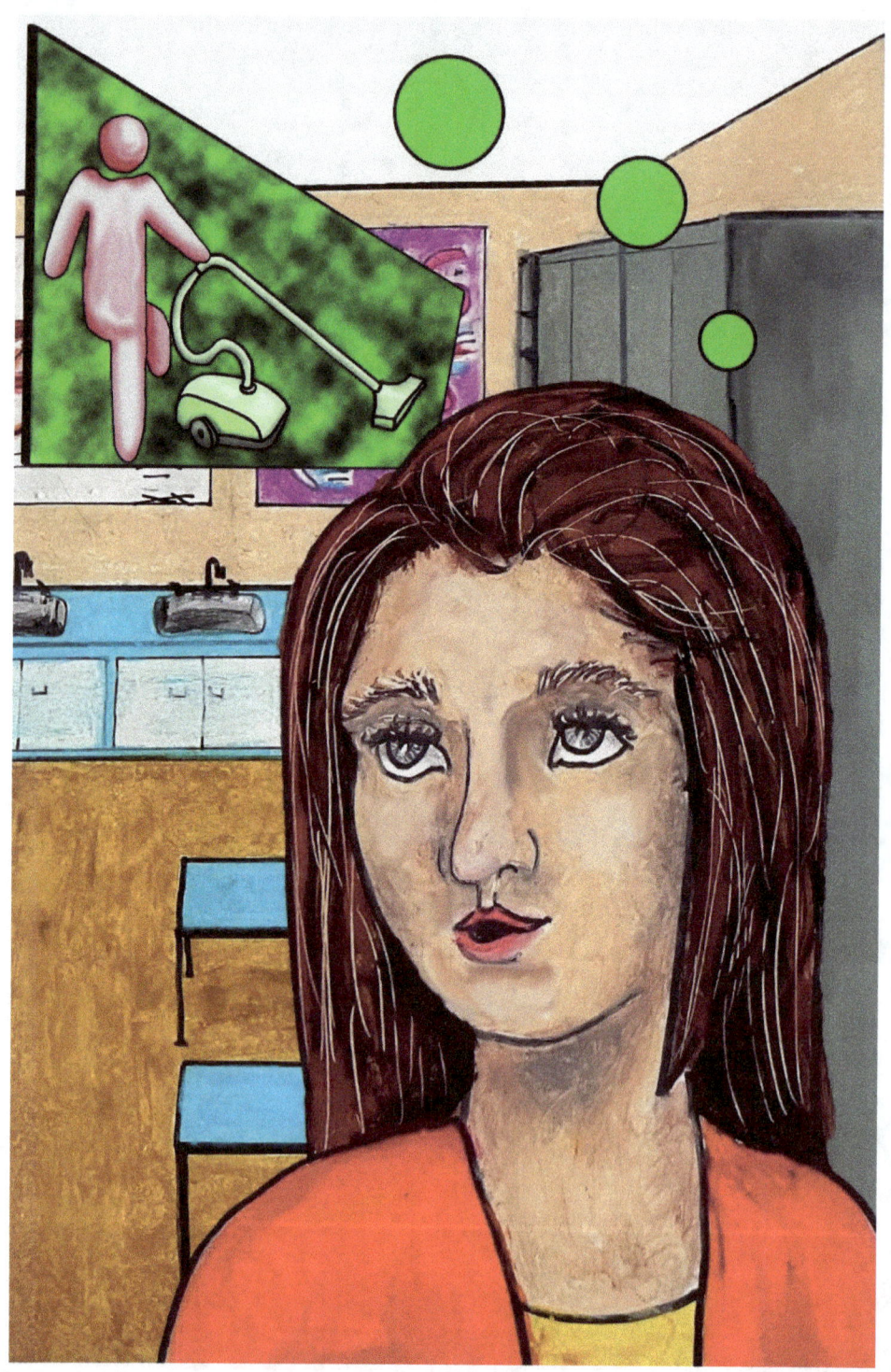

Awira raises her hand, and Nurse Dorothea calls on her to talk. "I use my anger and frustration to clean things. It helps me get out my negative energy and makes me productive at the same time. After I'm through cleaning, I'm relaxed and just want to sit down and enjoy a nice cup of lemonade."

"Using the energy of anger to motivate us to make our world better is an important skill that we must all learn to help society get to the place it needs to be, where everyone can find their place and live a fulfilling life," says Nurse Dorothea.

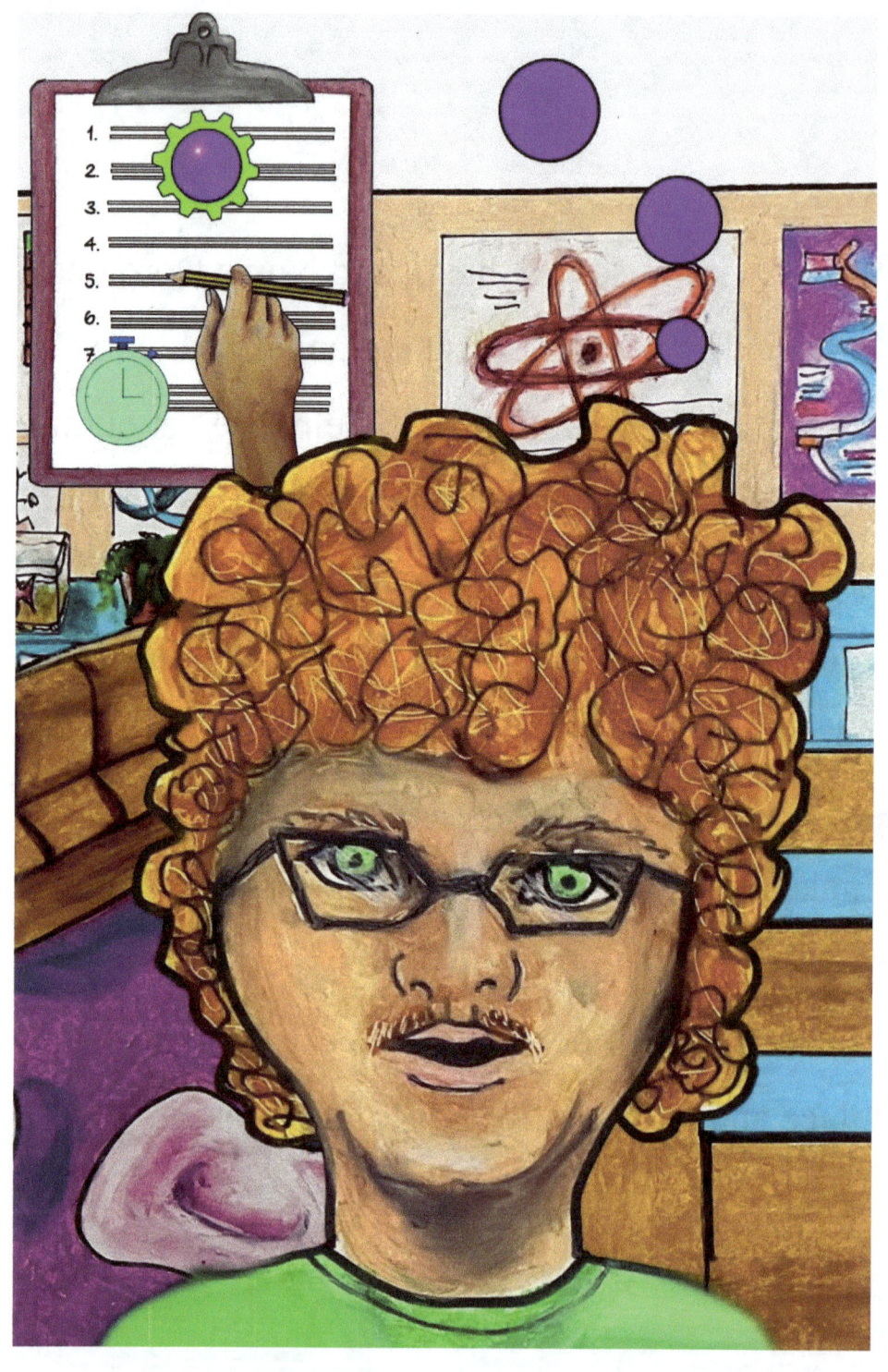

Connor raises his hand, and Nurse Dorothea calls on him to talk. "I use my anger energy to organize things. Once, I totally reorganized my closet. It helped distract my mind and process the energy. It also gave me time to think about the best response to the situation."

"Sometimes doing boring things can help give our mind the freedom to think about the best courses of action," says Nurse Dorothea.

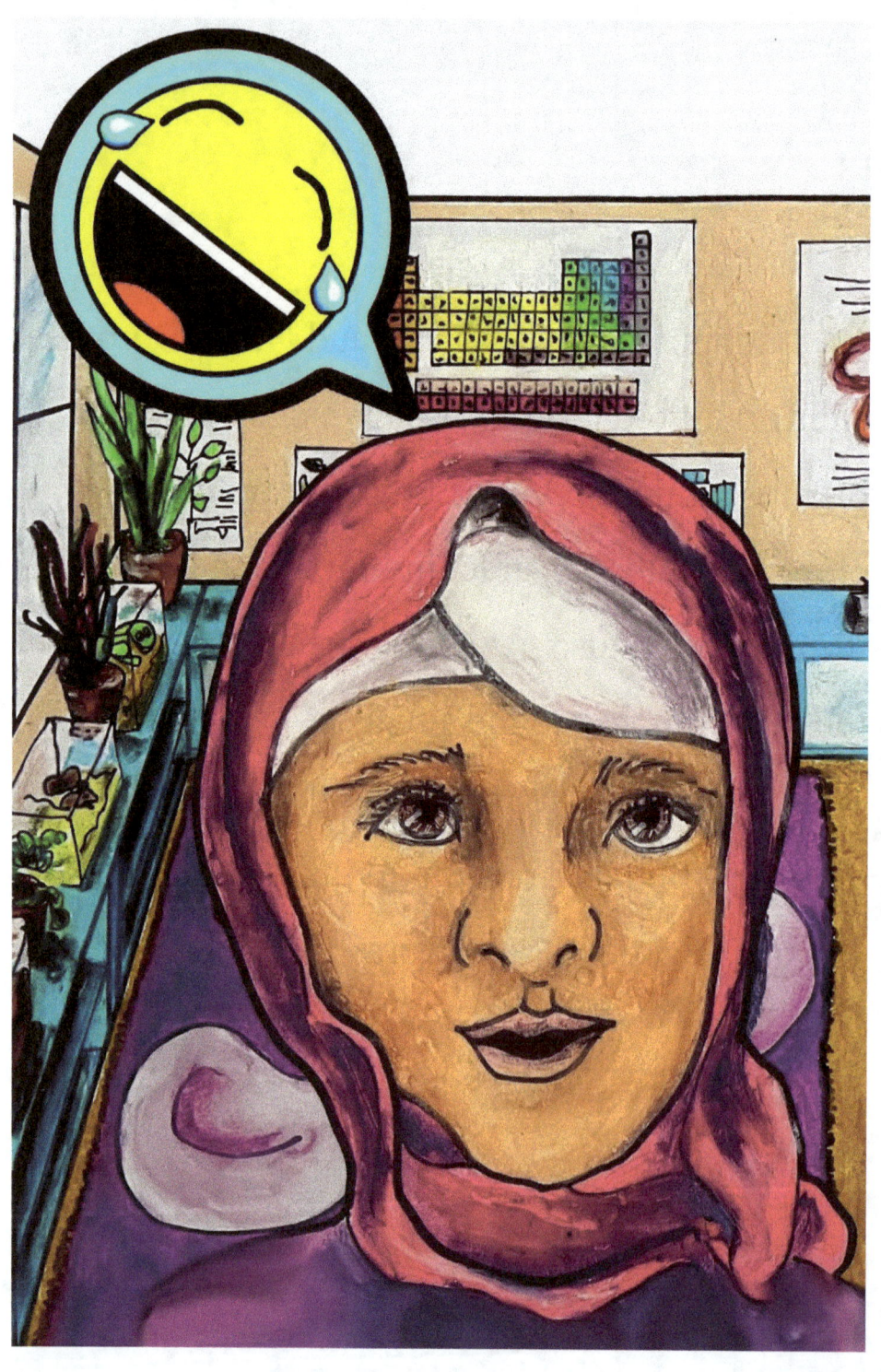

Fatima raises her hand, and Nurse Dorothea calls on her to talk. "I choose to use humor to respond to my anger. I guess it changes my emotions, and that's why it helps."

"That's exactly why some people are sarcastic. They choose humor to deal with their frustration so that the anger doesn't get too strong," says Nurse Dorothea.

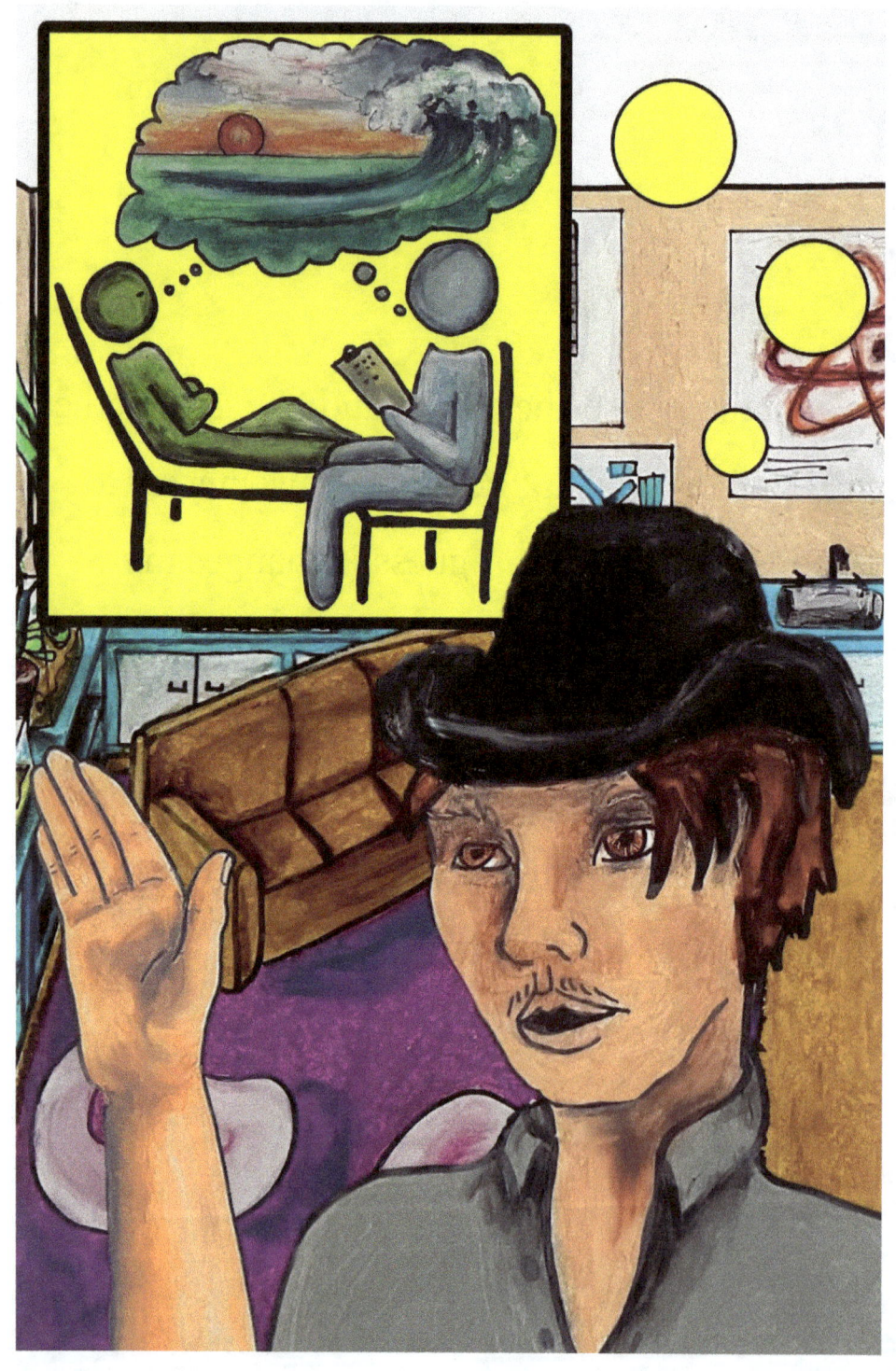

Wyatt raises his hand, and Nurse Dorothea calls on him to talk. "I saw a therapist once, and they did guided imagery to help me get through an angry emotion. They helped me visualize myself sitting on the beach relaxing. It helped me to switch emotions so that we could talk about things."

"Guided imagery is an effective coping skill for some people. It is best that the person has already experienced the place in the guided imagery, so they have something to relate to. You don't want to ask someone to imagine they are in a forest if they have only lived in a desert all their life," says Nurse Dorothea.

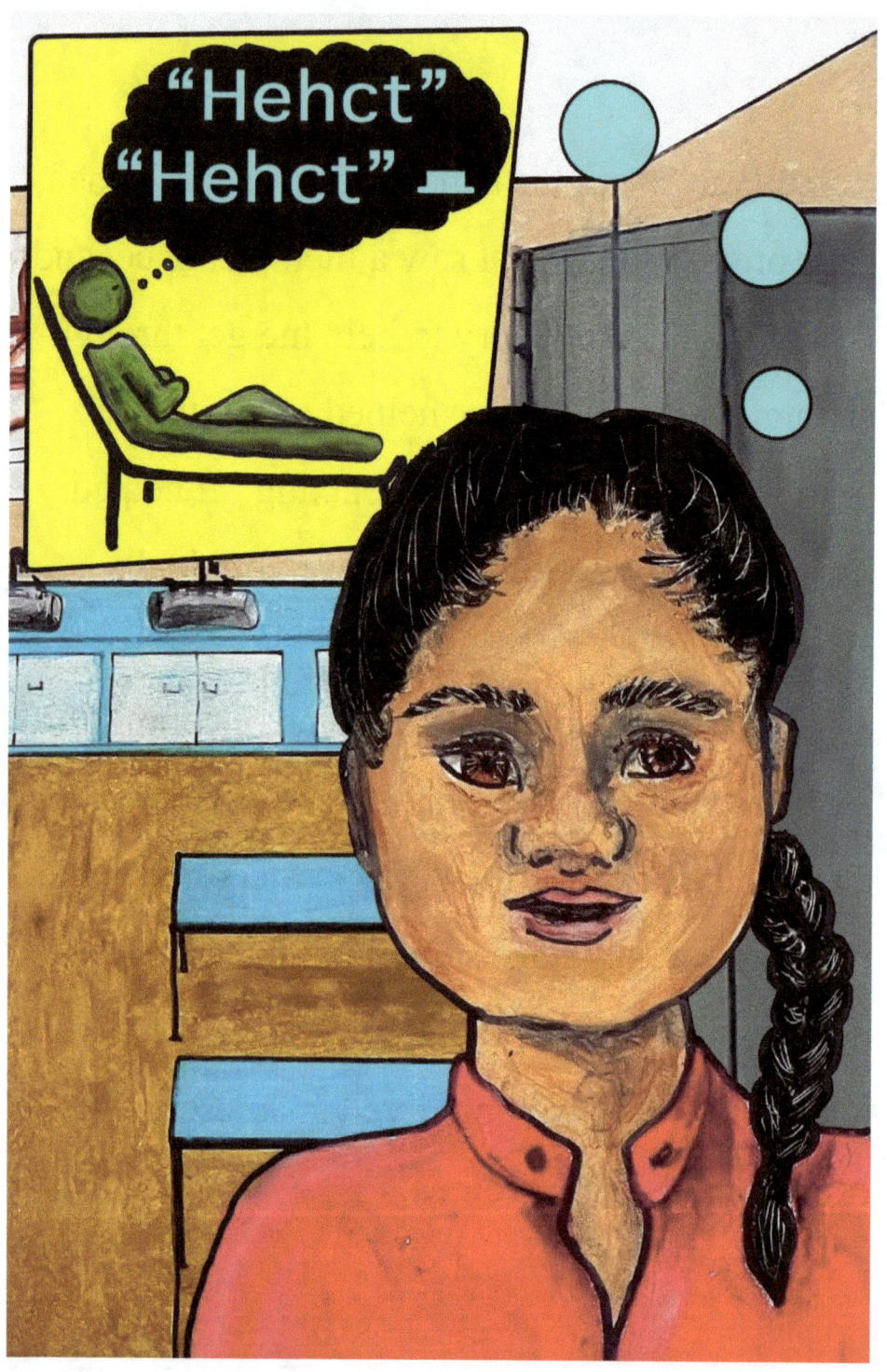

Pia raises her hand, and Nurse Dorothea calls on her to talk. "I've repeated the word relax over and over again, and it helped me relax when I was frustrated."

"Repeating something over and over again can help the mind focus on a place of being where you want to be so that you arrive there. It is like using positive affirmations," says Nurse Dorothea.

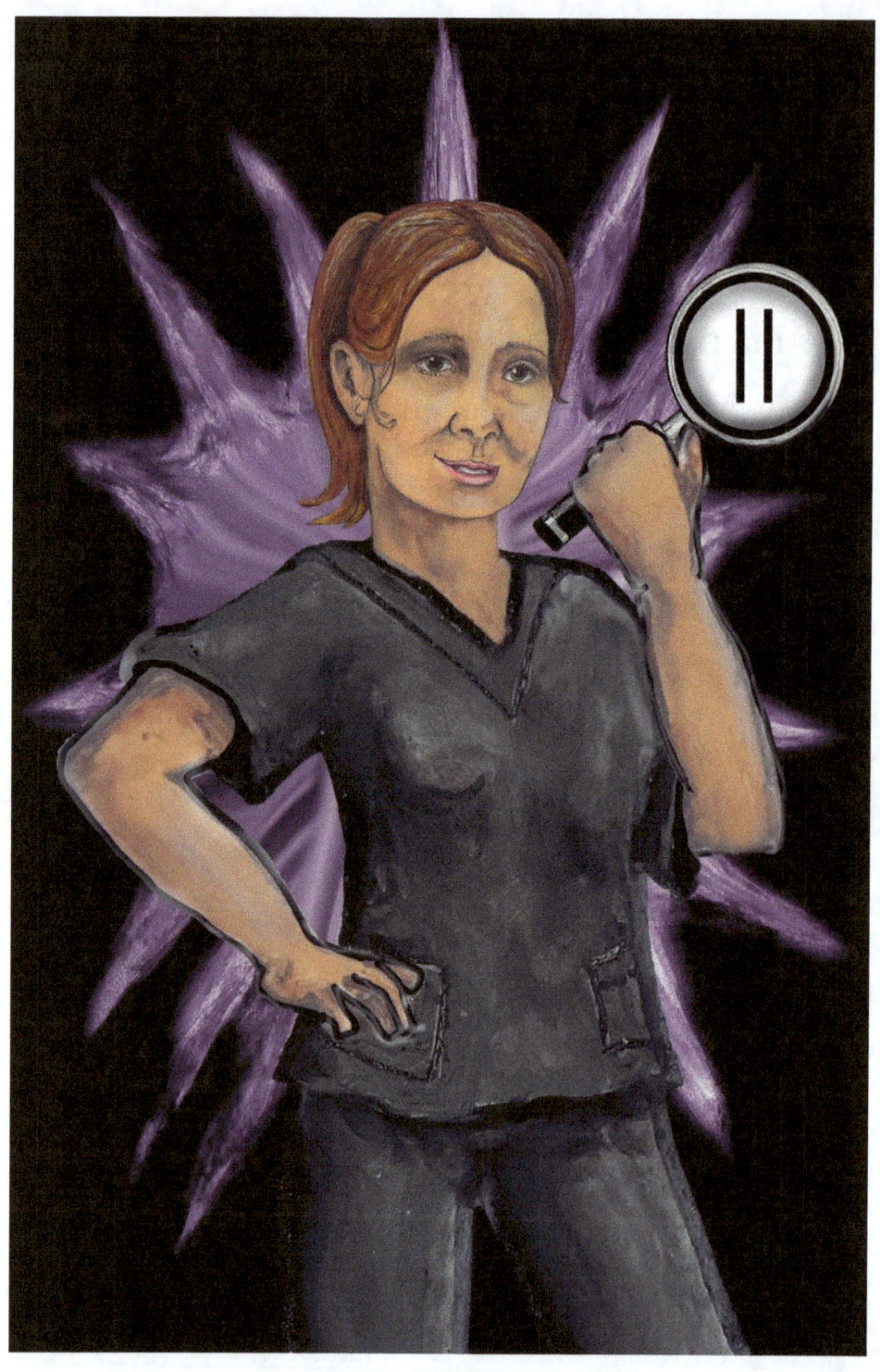

"We have gone over a lot of things, so let's take a short break and refresh ourselves. Those of you watching the video or reading the book, continue to do the lesson whenever you are ready. We'll see each other shortly."

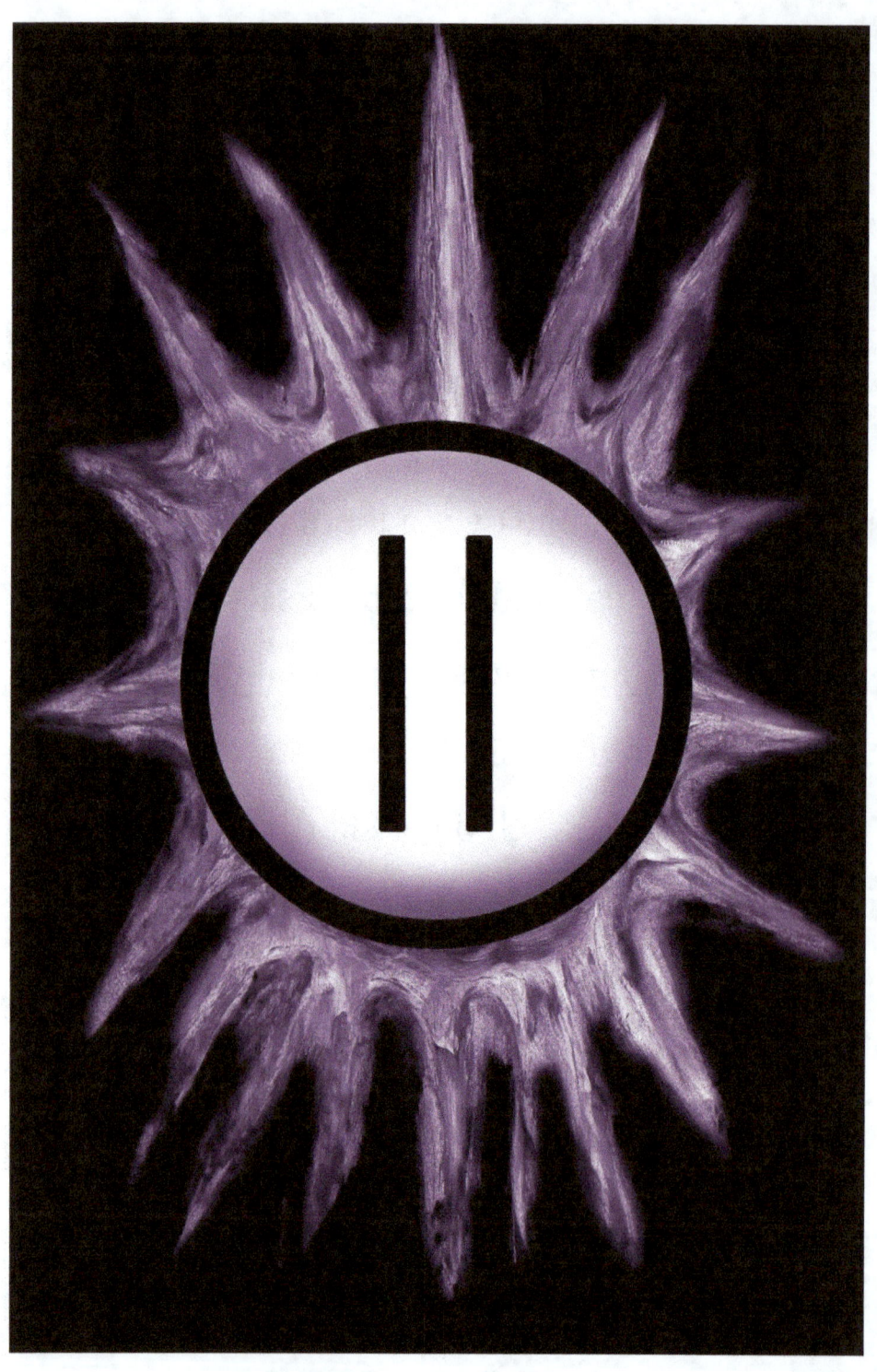

Part 3

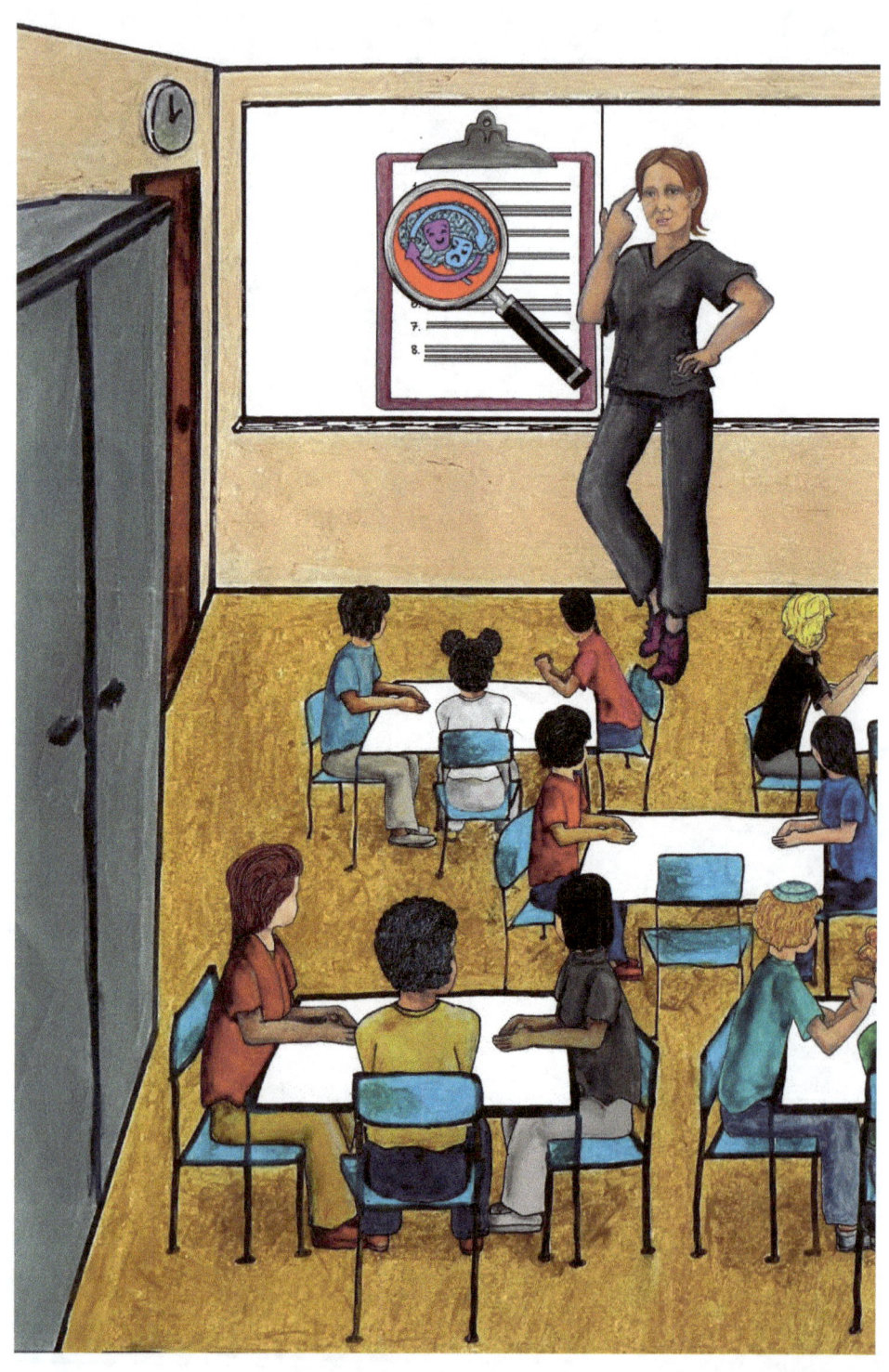

"Welcome back. When trying to manage your anger, you must first learn your triggers. Triggers for anger are things, people, or situations that cause anger to be created. *Merriam-Webster* defines trigger as something to cause an intense and usually negative emotional reaction in someone. There are some things you should learn about your triggers. You should learn what exactly the trigger is for your anger. You should learn how often the trigger occurs and if anger is always manifested when the trigger happens. You should learn the intensity of your anger with each trigger and observe your feelings. You should learn how you tend to react to each trigger. Some triggers may cause you to be verbally aggressive, and other triggers may cause you to brood and perseverate about the incident. Even seeing a person could be a trigger."

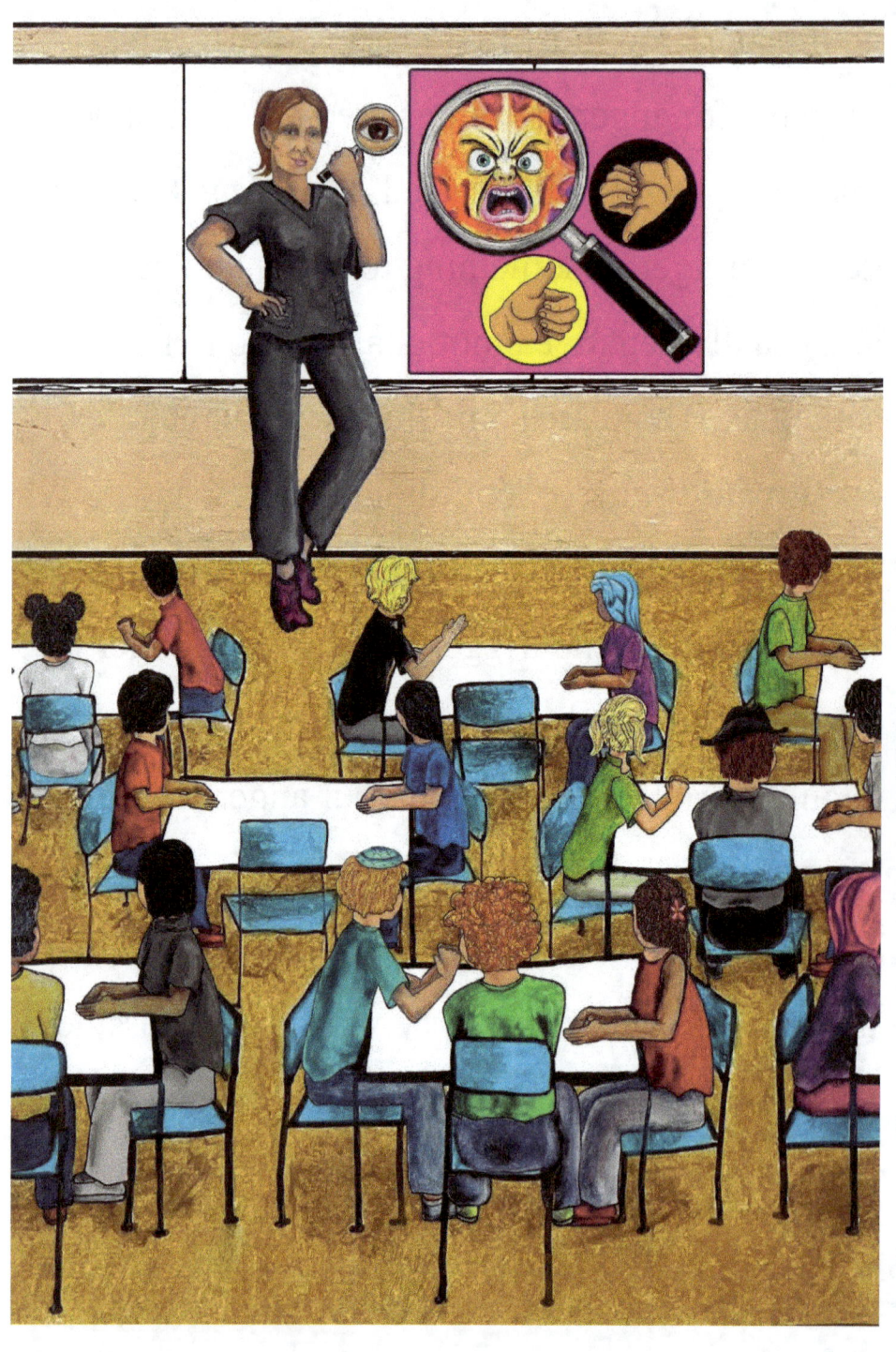

"You should examine if your anger is helpful or unhelpful. In some situations, anger can be helpful because it can be a survival mechanism. In other situations, your anger and how you react to it may be unhelpful because you may exaggerate your response and do something in excess which can cause relationships to be broken. You should avoid burning bridges or breaking relationships because you never know when you might need the person in your life. Burning bridges should be used for extreme circumstances and should not be the normal thing to do since it can cause a person to be alone without support."

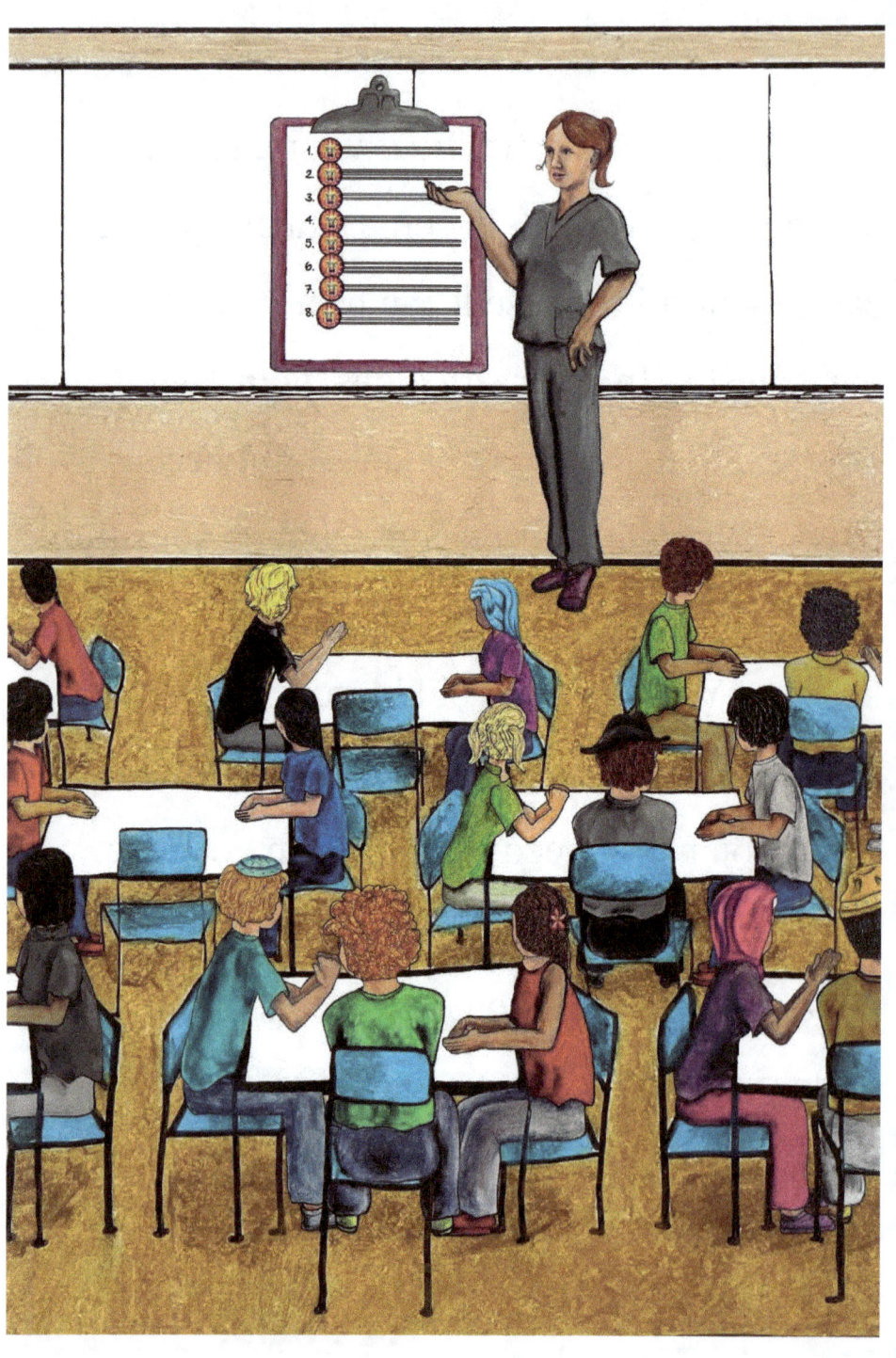

"To help identify your triggers, you can start by listing the things that make you angry. Try to be as detailed as possible, since a person may not necessarily make you angry, but what the person says or how they say it may be the reason that you get angry. Try to think with complexity, since your anger may be triggered by abstract ideas like social injustice. List all the things, people, situations, events, and other things that may cause your anger. Doing this could be therapeutic by itself."

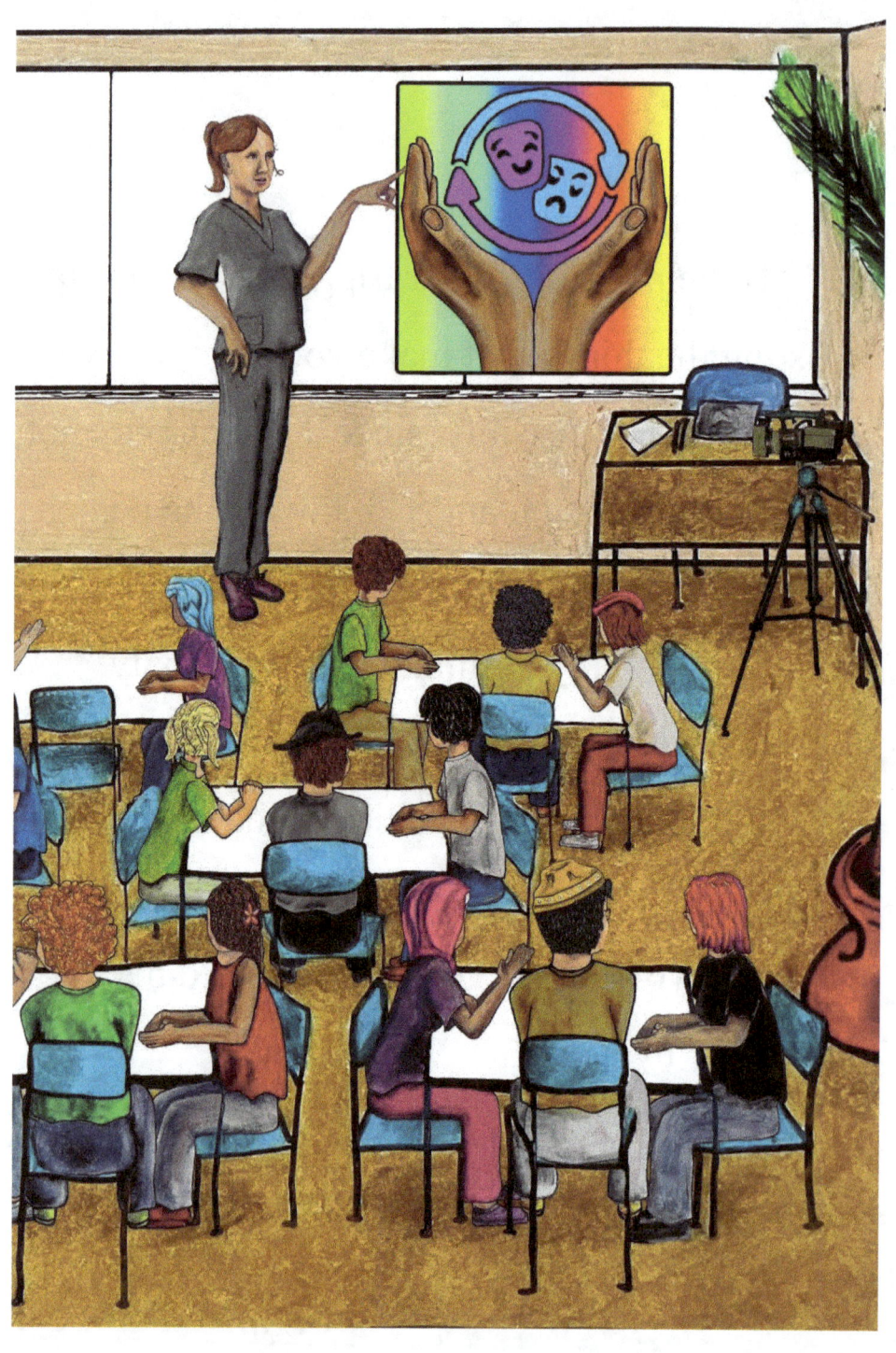

"You should also try to understand your underlying emotions. Emotions can be seen on a spectrum where one emotion could easily lead to another. Someone's depression could lead to anger. Someone may have developed the skill of forgiveness, so that anger leads to forgiveness, which then leads to peace and tranquility. Understanding all your emotions is part of the key to managing anger since it can be such a strong emotion."

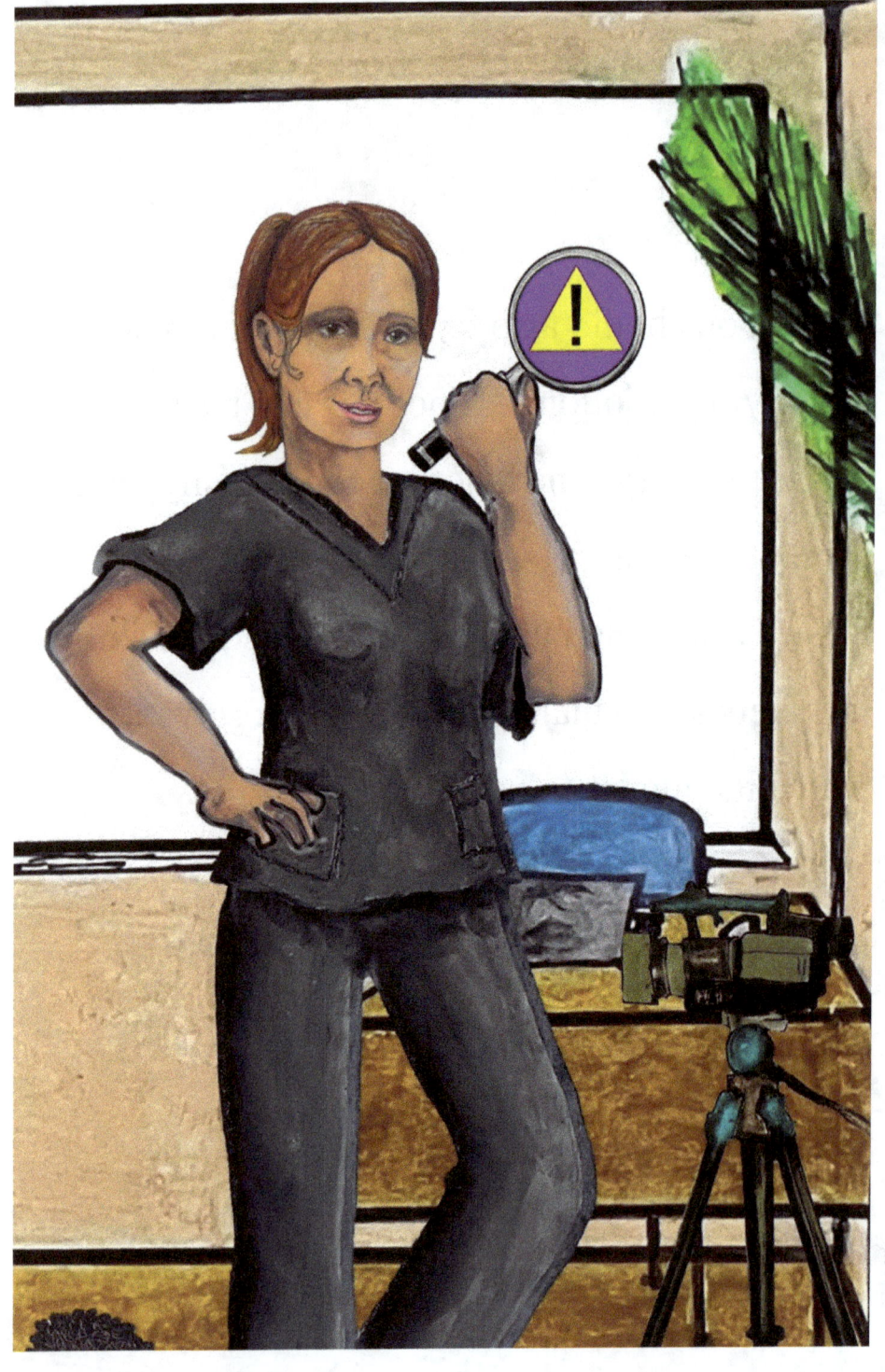

"After you have listed your triggers for anger, list your warning signs that people can observe from you, which would show that you're getting angry. Some people clinch their fists. Some people frown and grimace. Some people start yelling. Some people might start pacing around the room or down a hallway. Everyone is unique, and how a person responds to anger could be unique in their own way. Understanding yourself and how you react is another key to managing anger."

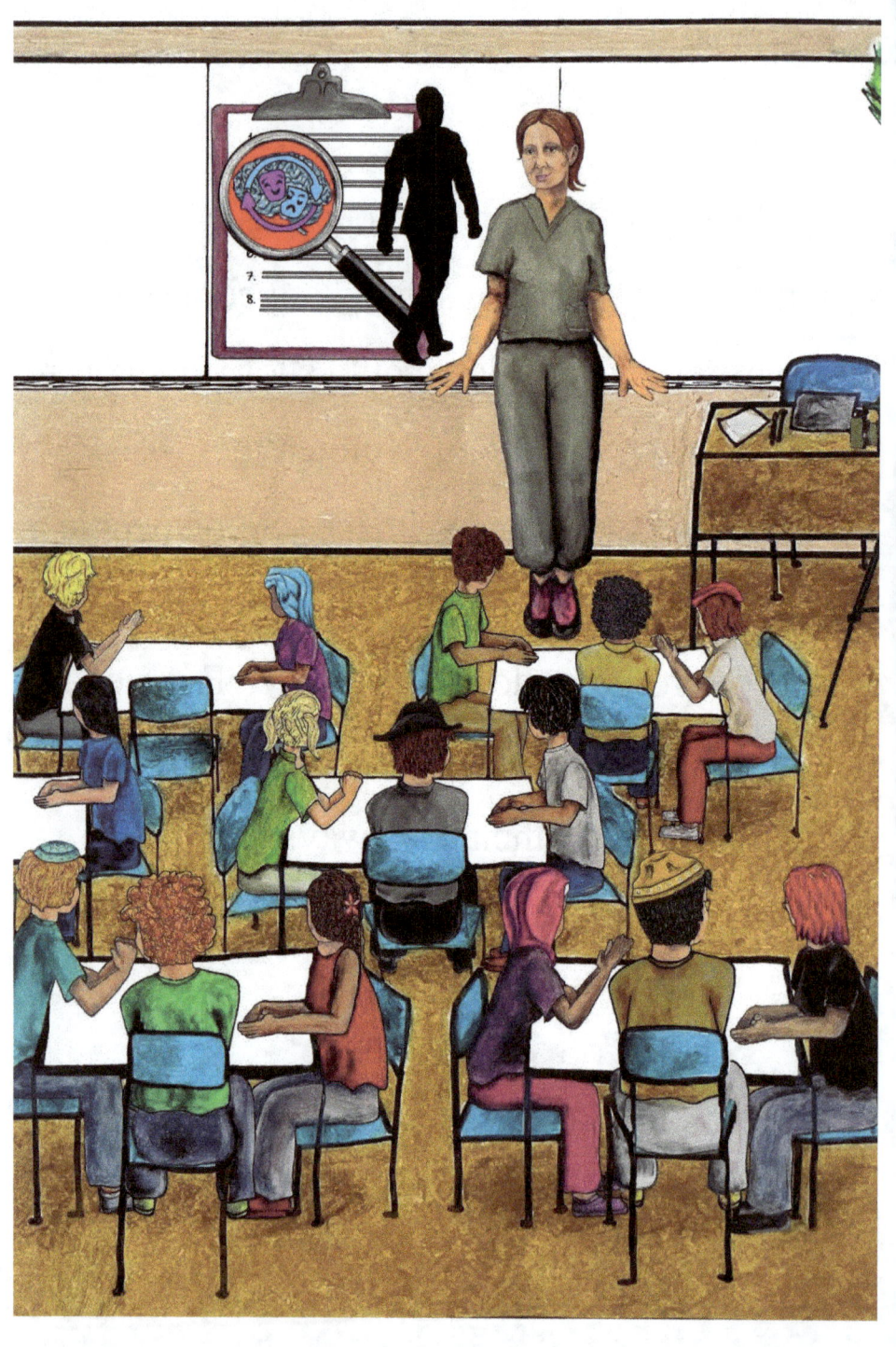

"Once you learn your triggers and warning signs, you can learn to step away from the person or situation if needed, so that the anger doesn't easily escalate into verbal or physical aggression. Stepping away to give distance between you and the trigger can help you manage anger before it gets so strong that it starts to manage you. You can make a list of things someone can do to help you with your warning signs. When there are warning signs, it is time to do something to de-escalate your anger before you act out. Some may choose to read a religious text, play a game, visit their happy place in their mind, or take prescribed medication. The point is to do something to prevent a situation from escalating."

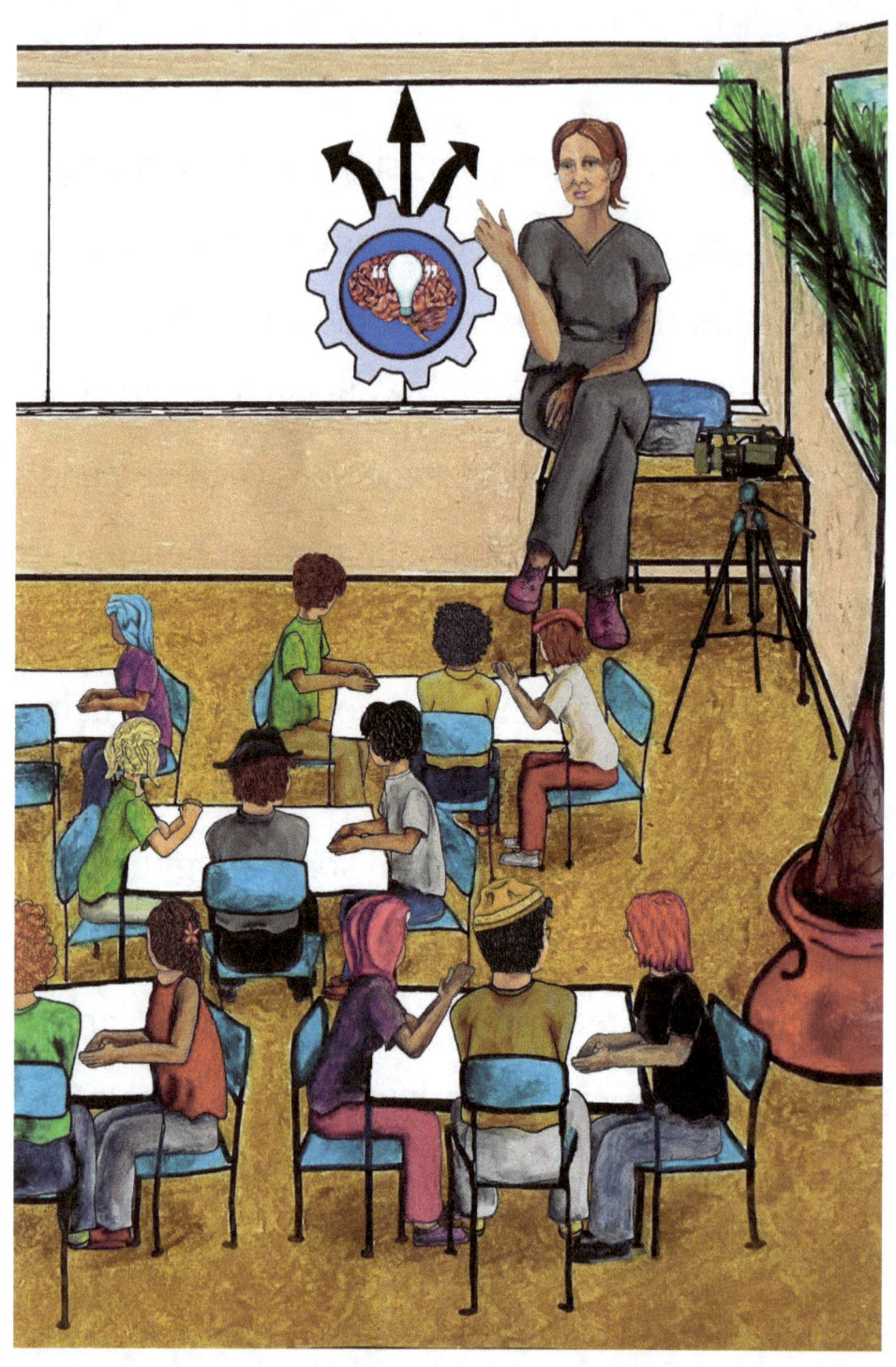

"Consider alternative thinking to manage your anger. Think about your thinking. Think about what you were thinking when you got angry, and if the thoughts were valid. If you were thinking that you knew what someone else was thinking, consider that you may not have any ability to understand other people's thoughts, and that it may be a false belief to believe you hear other people's thoughts. The brain is a powerful organ and can help you believe things that are not true. We must face our thoughts with courage and realize that initial beliefs may be false. It takes courage to tell yourself that you may not know the truth about something. Ask yourself what the facts of the situation are. Be a good observer and do your best to dig for the truth. Ask yourself if the thoughts are realistic or rational. Ask yourself what thoughts would be more realistic."

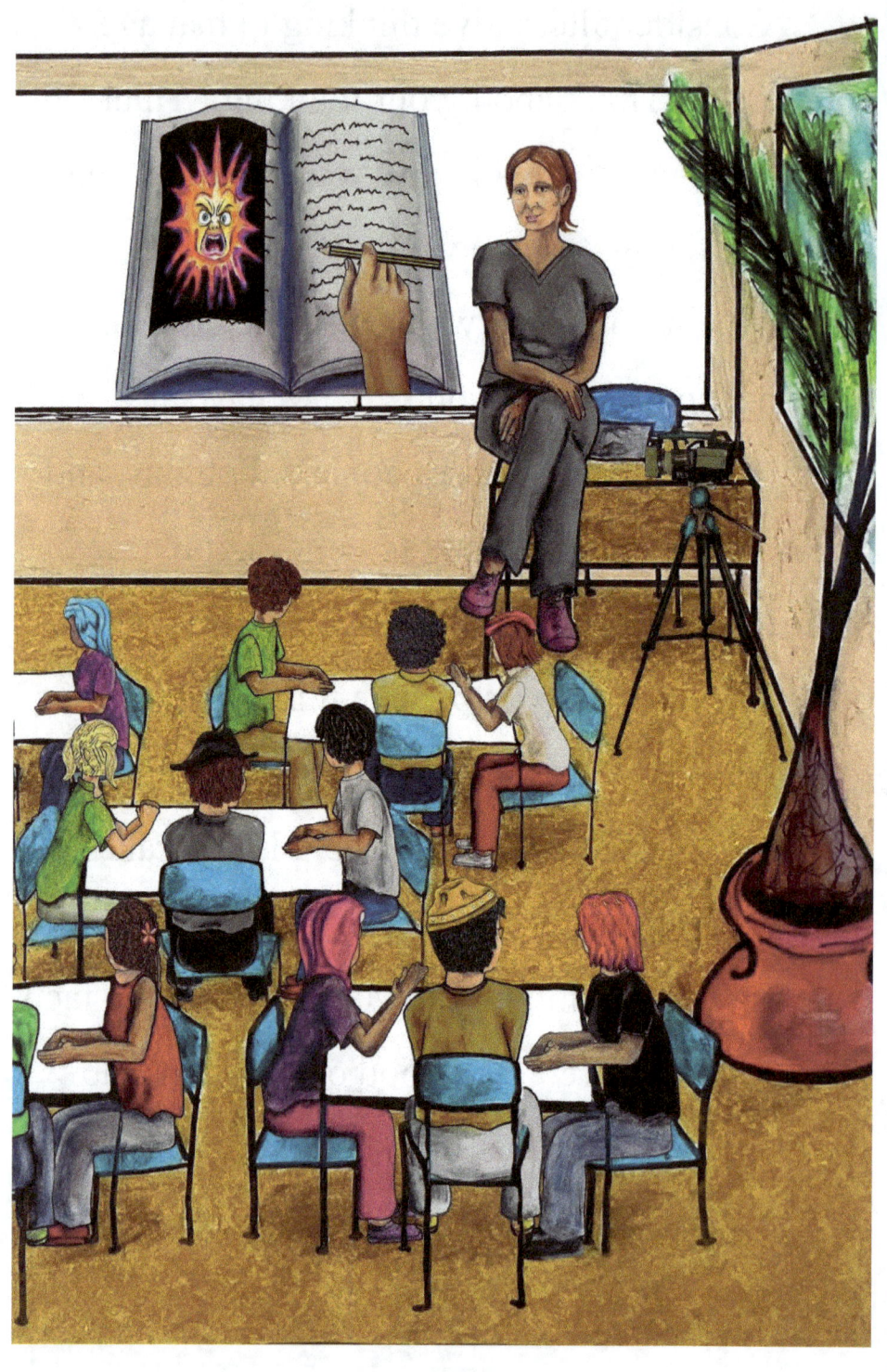

"If you struggle with anger, an idea worth practicing is keeping an anger diary. This is where each page in the diary is meant to describe the situation that caused anger, how you responded, what your warning signs for the event were, and how you tried to manage your anger. This will help you see what works for you in managing your anger, so that you can be on a path of continuous improvement."

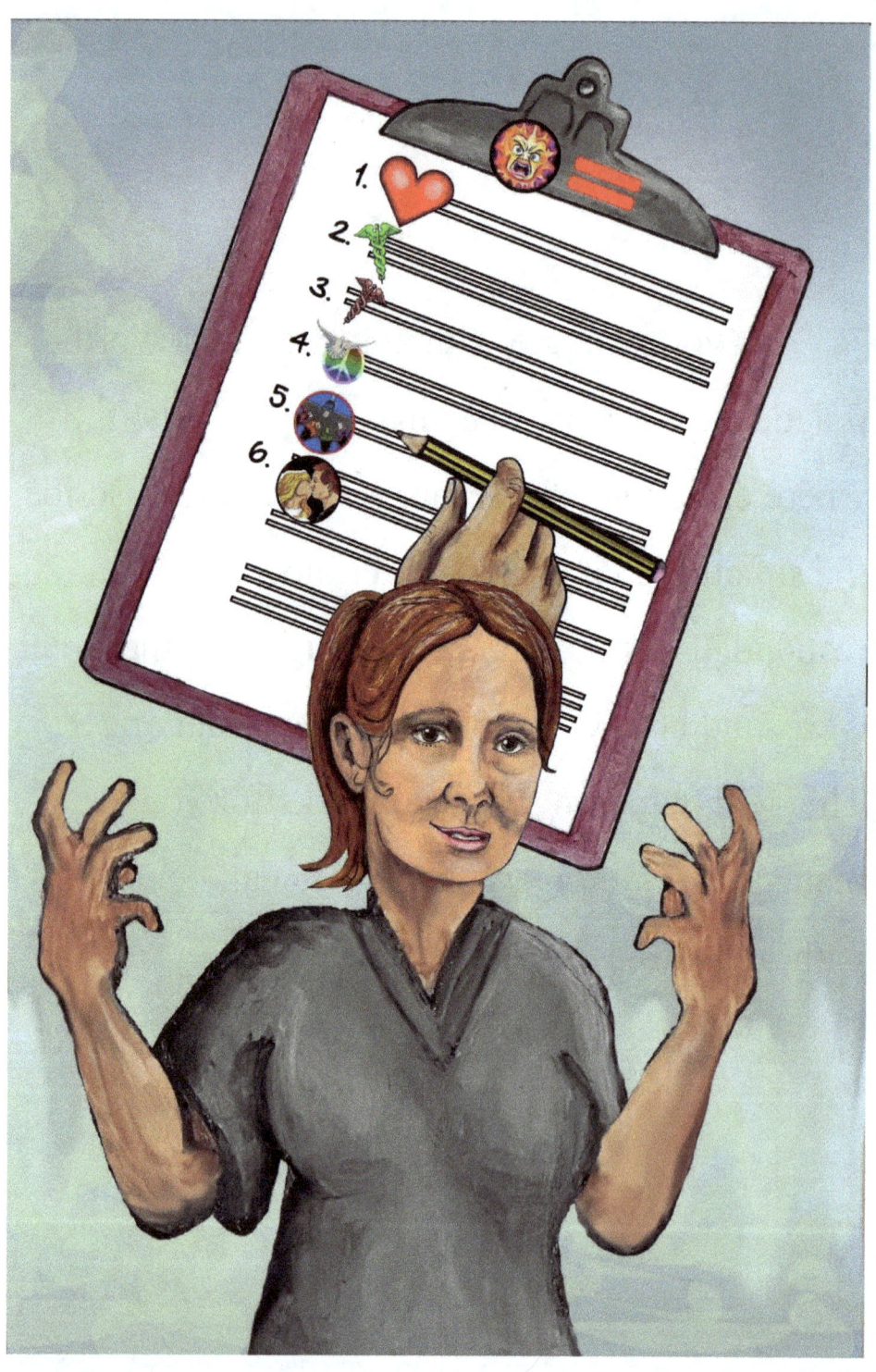

"Another helpful tip for your journey of anger management is to list things that are impacted by your anger. It could be relationships, employment, school, mental health, communication, plans for the future, and other things. Doing this will help you realize how impactful anger can be and can help motivate you to change and improve in your anger management skills."

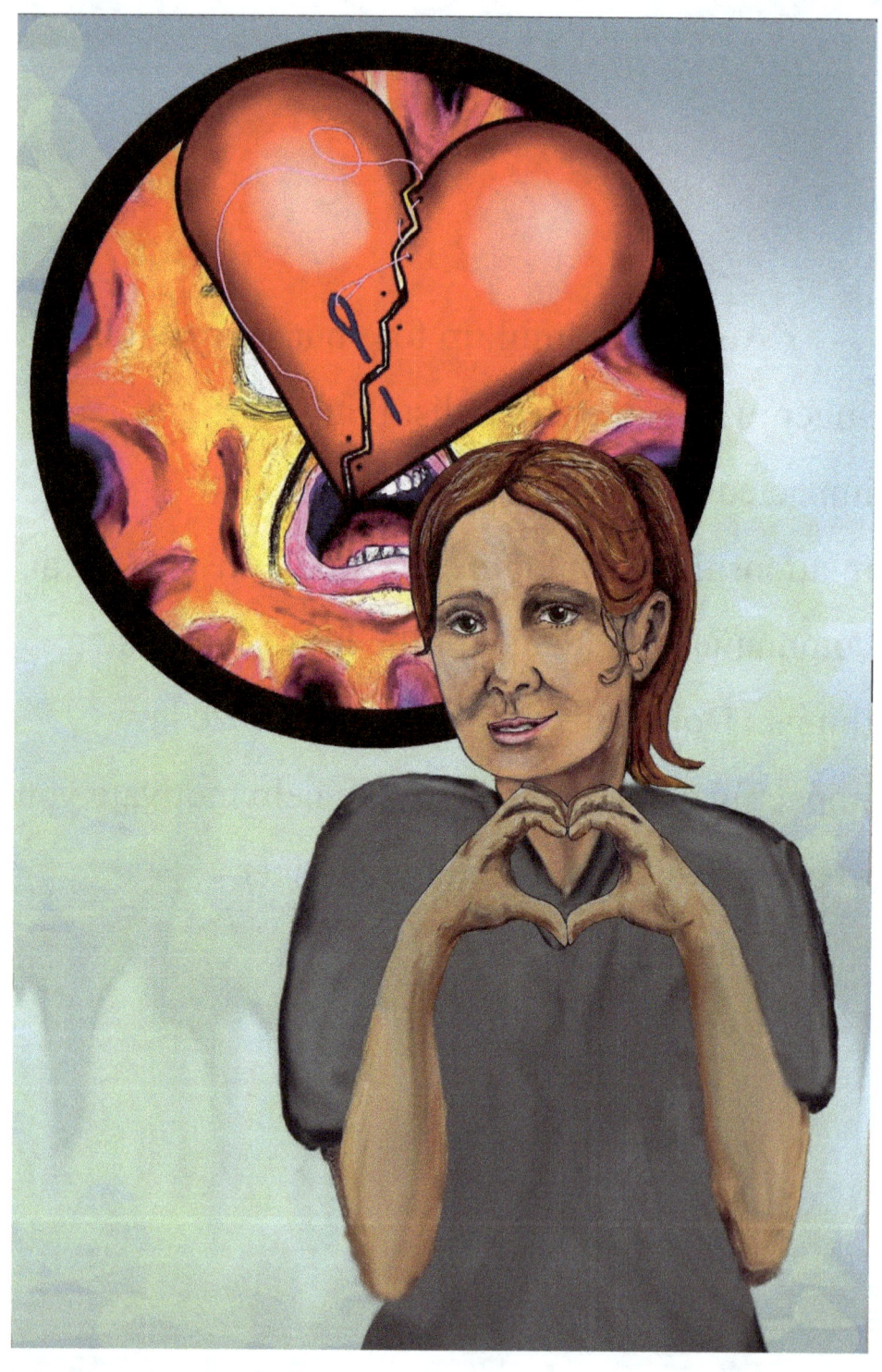

"When you have an angry outburst, you should offer to make amends. You should go to the people involved and tell them you are sorry and are on a journey of improvement. You should acknowledge that you have more work to do with anger management and hope they understand that it will take time to improve. You should offer to pay for and fix property that was damaged. You should offer to do something nice to show your regret. Doing something can make a difference."

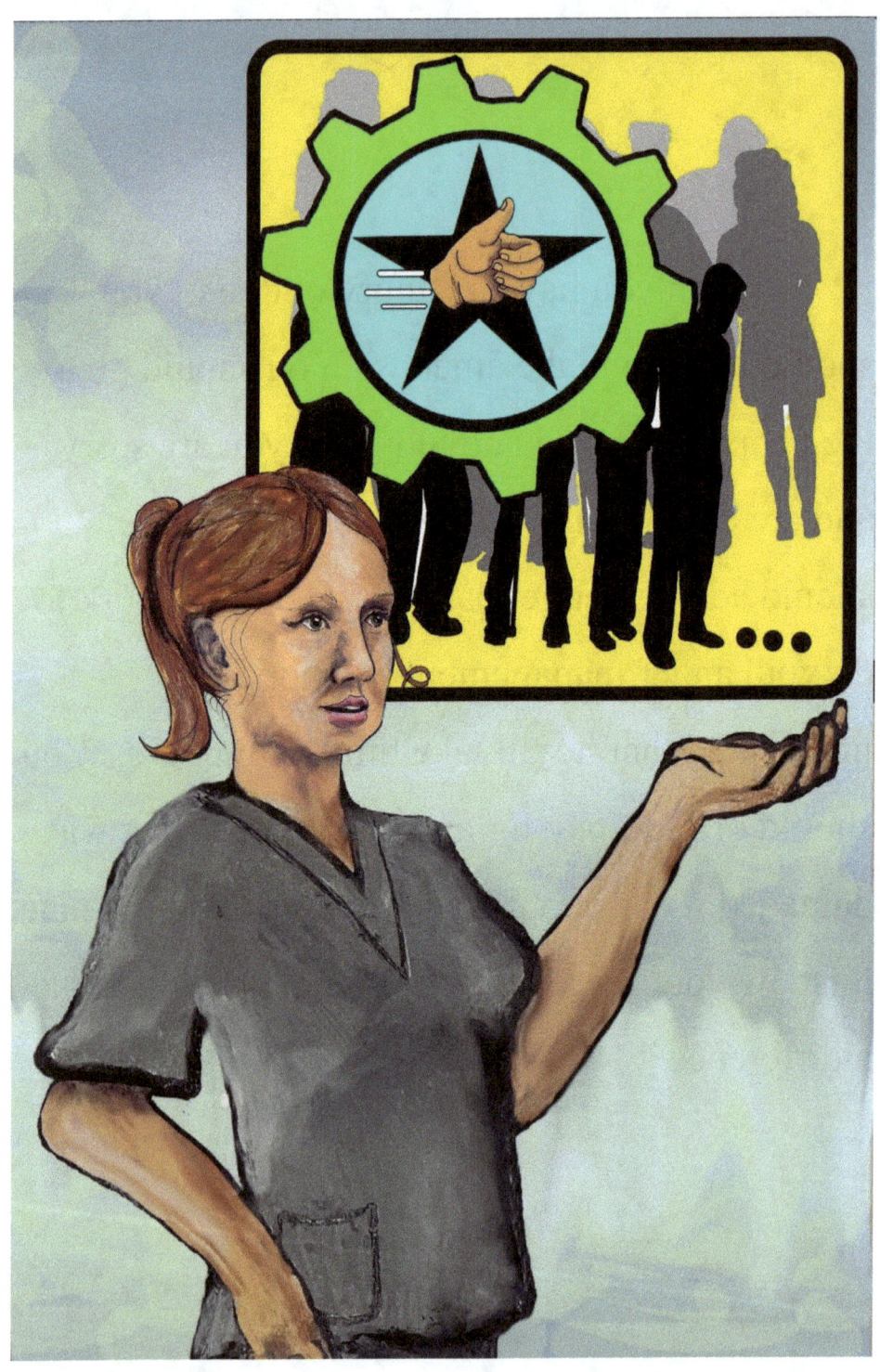

"Managing your expectations of others can also help with anger management. If you expect things from people or situations that are not possible, then it is easy to get frustrated and angry. I'm not saying to keep a low bar or very low expectations of everyone that you know so that you avoid frustration, but having realistic expectations of people and things can help avoid frustration which can lead to anger."

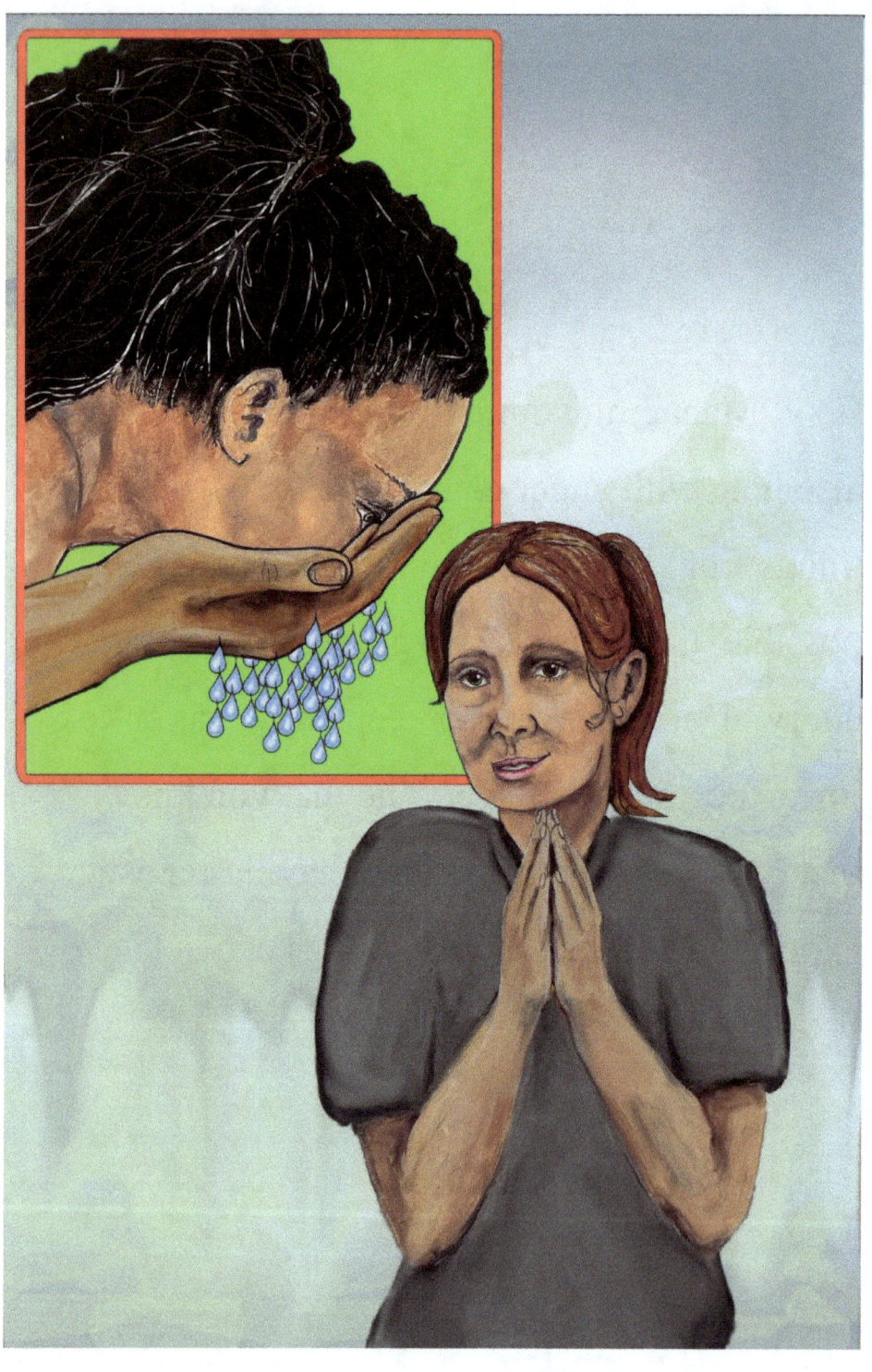

"If you get angry, one technique to help you calm down is putting cold water on your face. Try it the next time you are near a water faucet. Excuse yourself to use the bathroom. You won't know if it works until you try it."

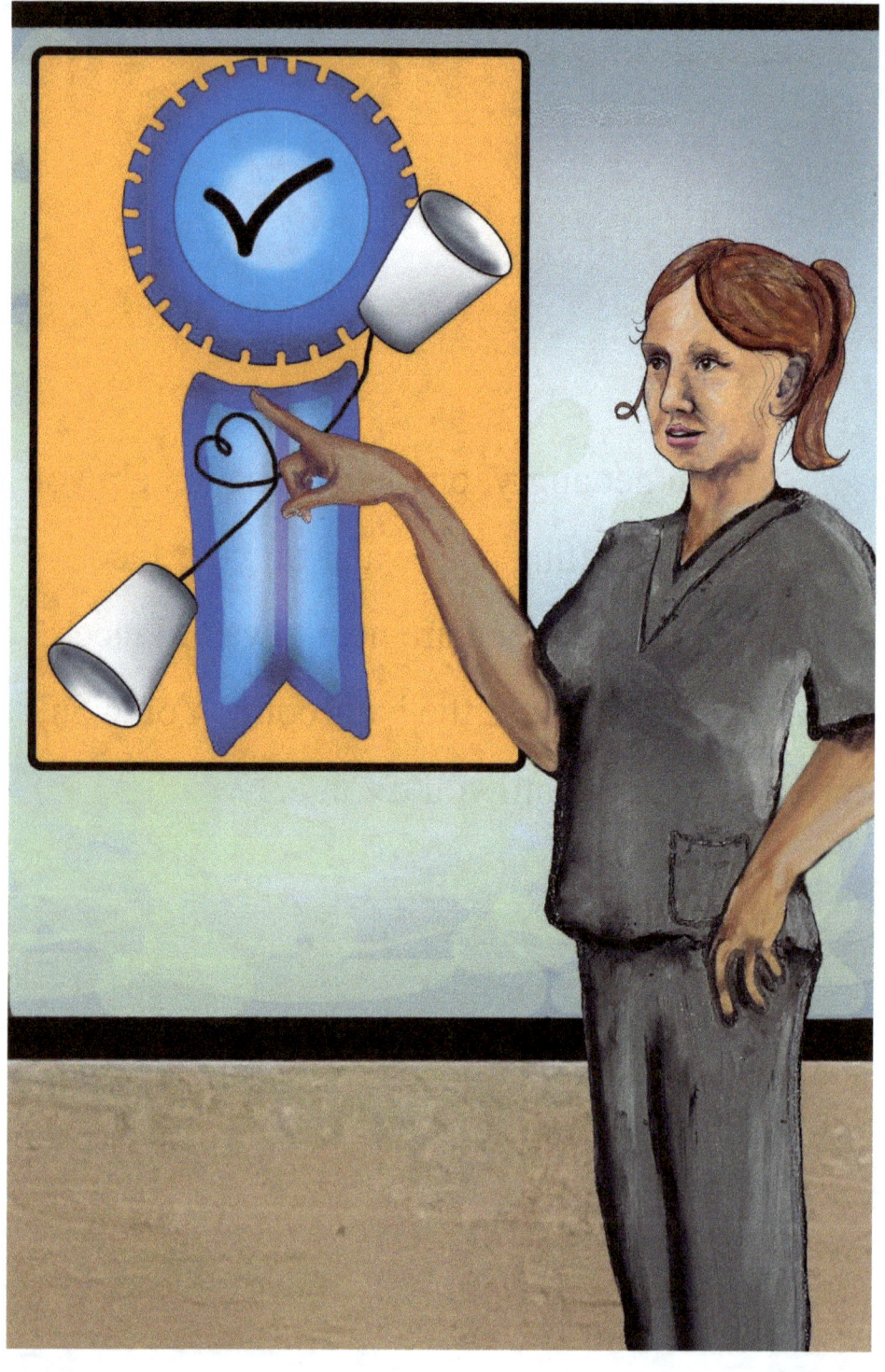

"Anger management requires good communication skills. Practice every day to say what you mean, mean what you say, and don't say it mean. Take a class on communication. Read a book about communication. Do things to increase your skills. Talk frequently with loved ones, so that your skills sharpen and stay sharpened. Good communication skills will not only help you with anger management, but also in other areas in life, such as employment and healthy relationships."

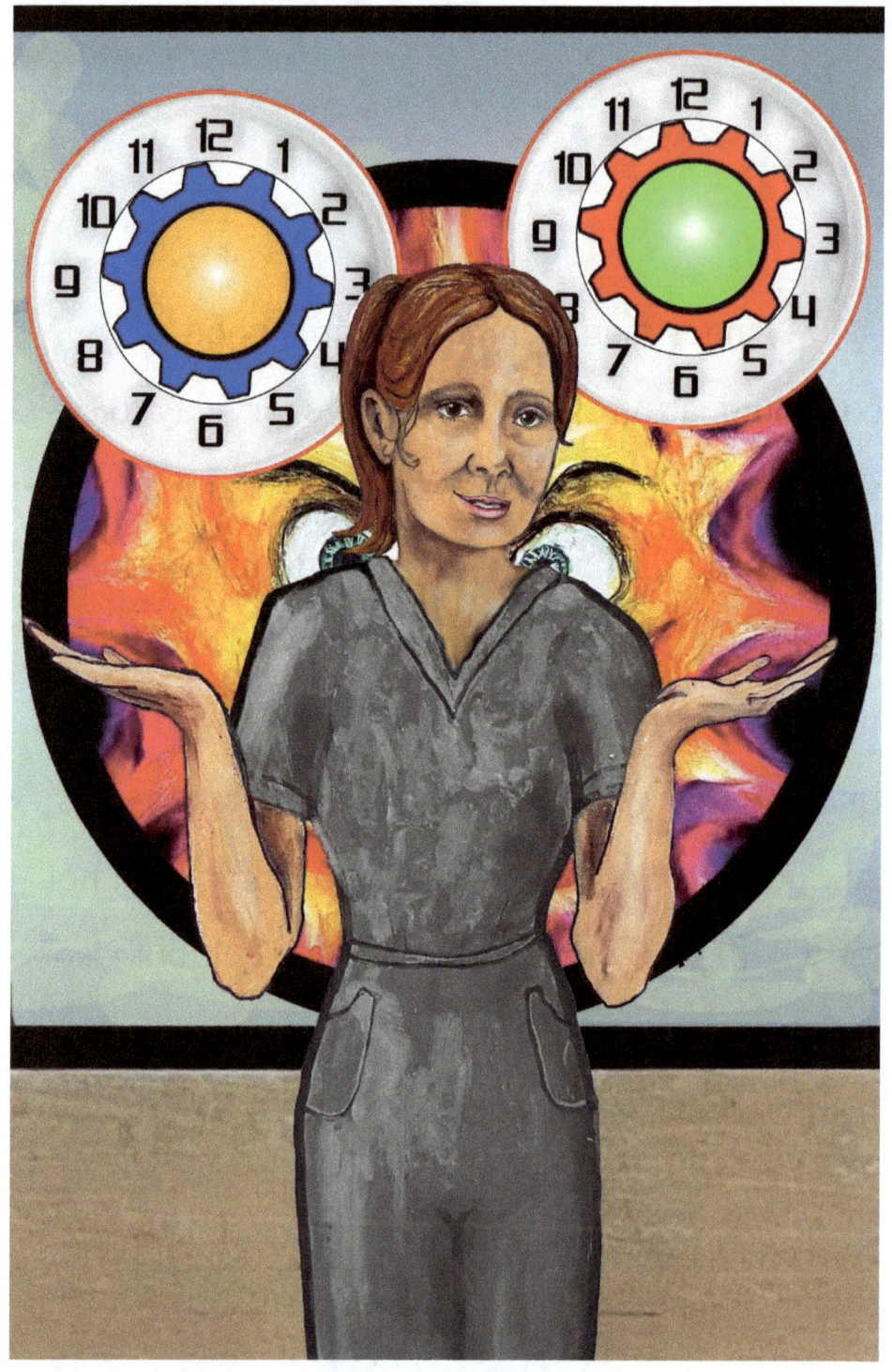

"Try changing the timing of things. If you notice you are always angry when you wake up, then try going to sleep earlier to get a better night's rest. You could try doing certain things at different times of the day if you notice you get angry when you do certain things in the evening. Change routines as needed so that you can manage things better."

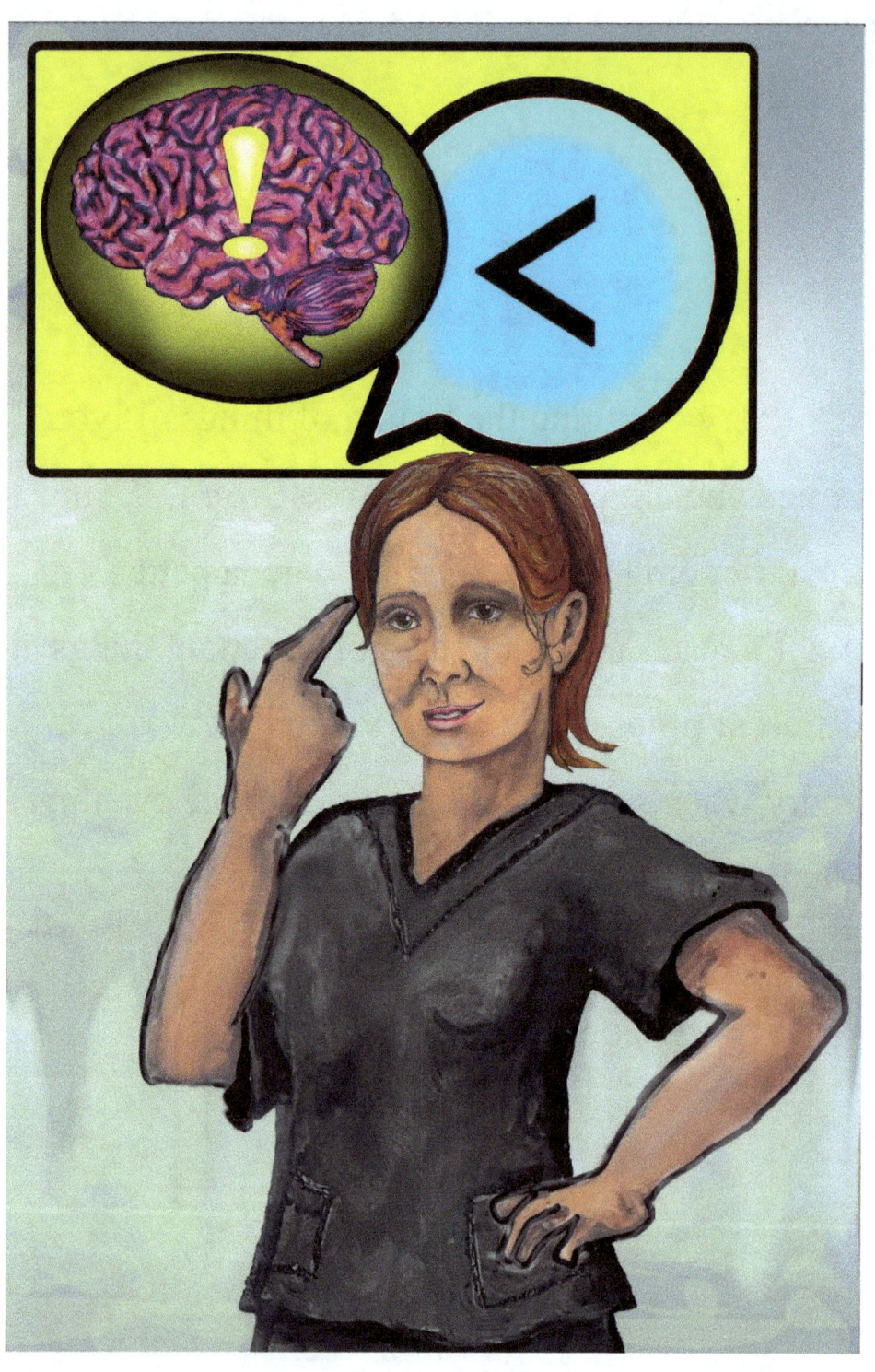

"Practice thinking before speaking. When you get angry, practice the skill of keeping silent for a short amount of time, so that you can carefully consider your response. This also counts for written communication like emails. You should never write an email out of anger and then send it. It's like talking out of anger without thinking about your words. Write your email, and save it in draft form. Come back to your email later that day or the next day, and evaluate if you should edit it. Usually, an angry email should not be sent."

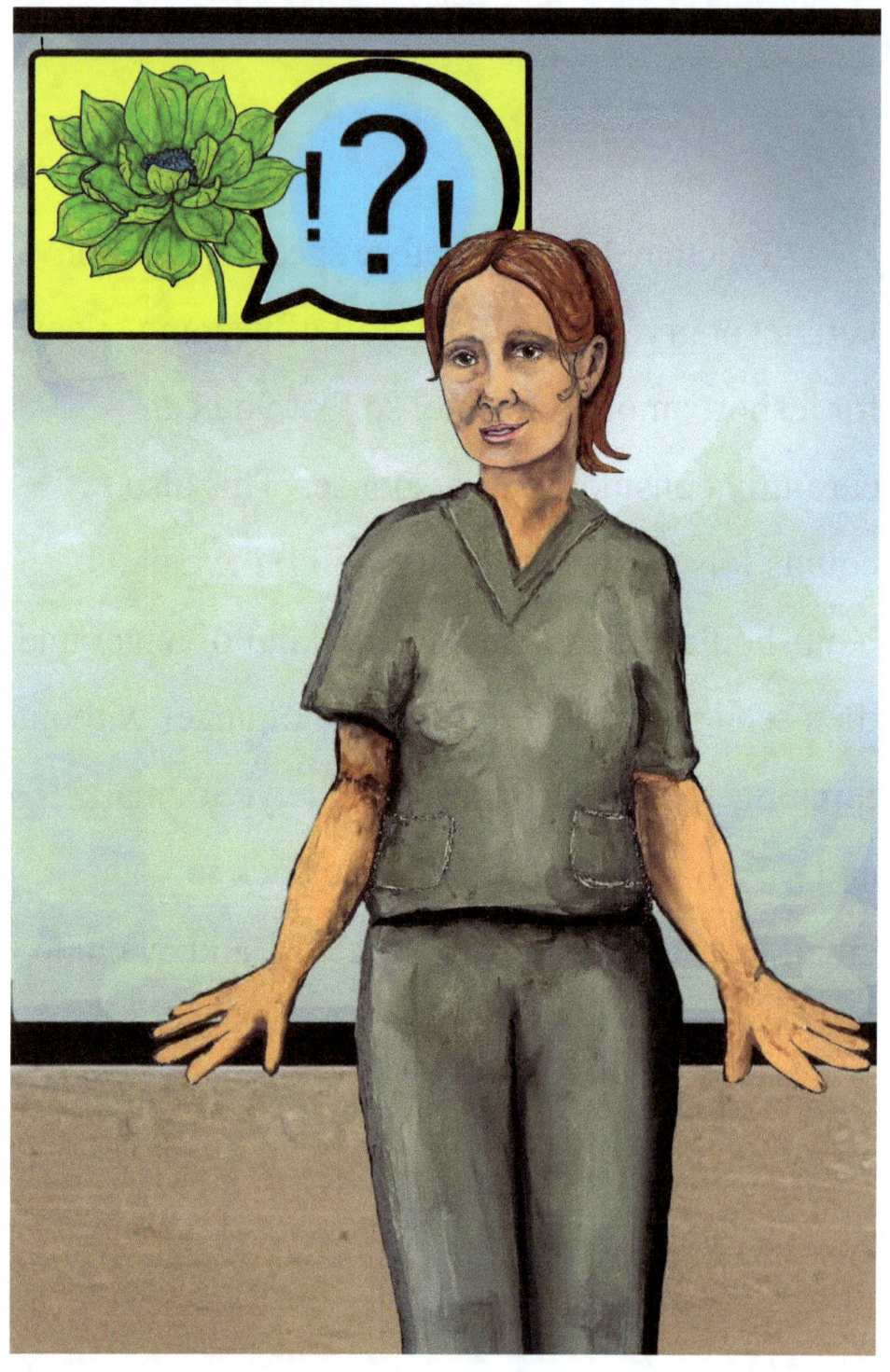

"After you have calmed down, express your concerns. If you express your concerns while you are angry, you may use a hostile tone of voice. That is why you should wait some time after the incident to express your concerns, so that you do it carefully and with a good approach."

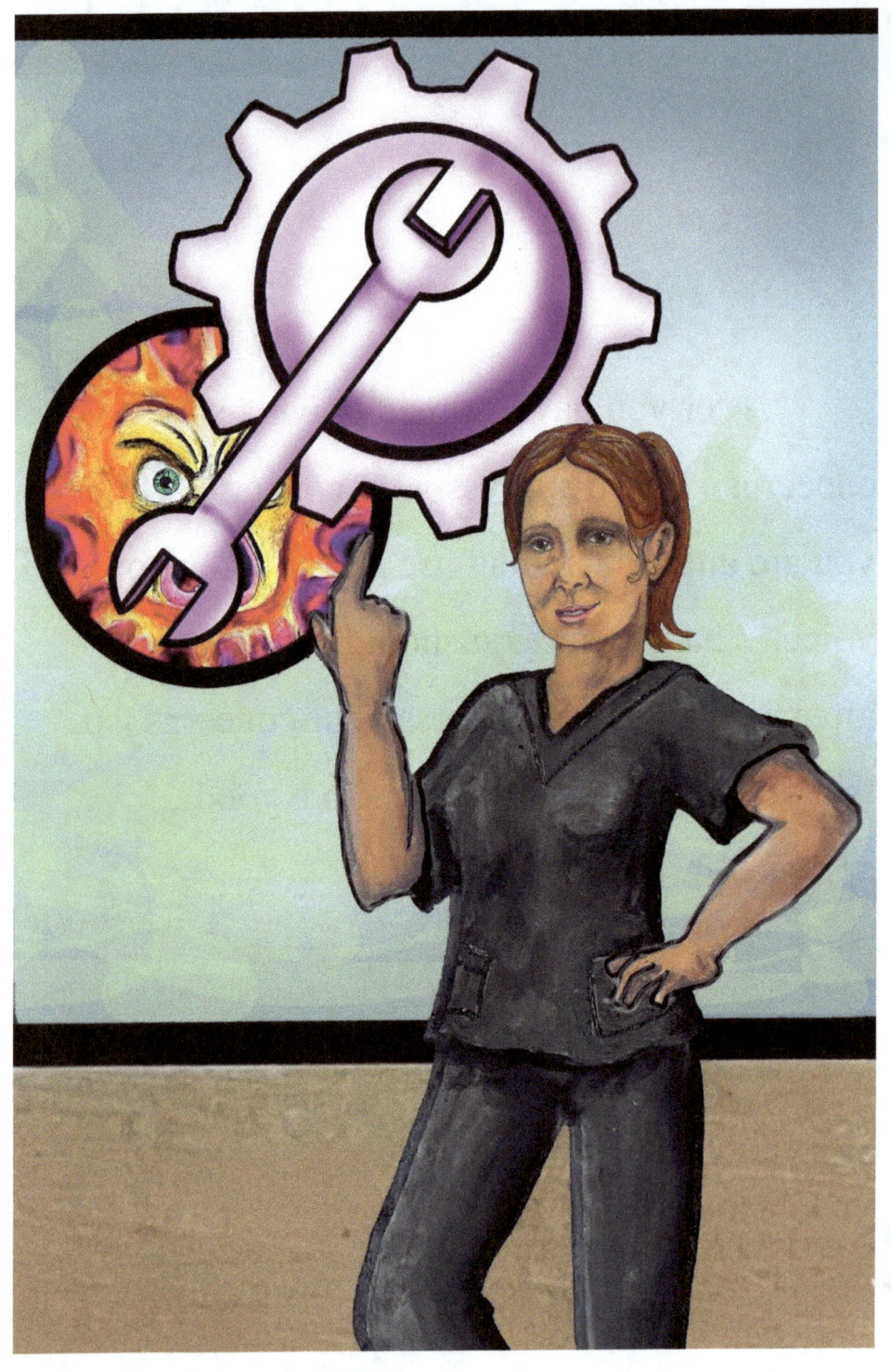

"Be a problem solver, and seek solutions to your anger. Avoid being angry just to be angry. Use your anger to drive yourself into action so that issues are resolved. Take action instead of just feeling the anger."

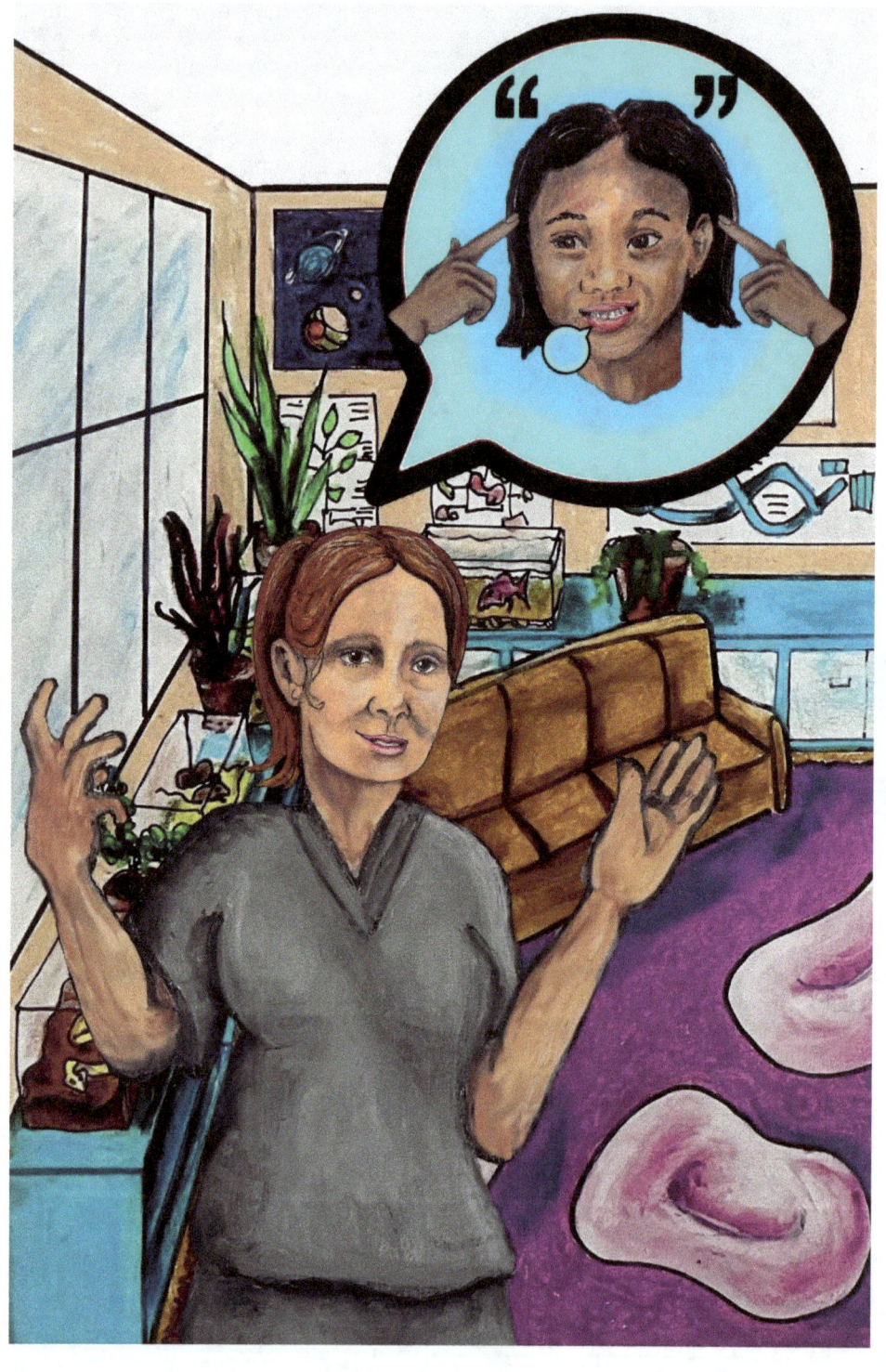

"When you discuss things that make you angry, use 'I' statements. Such as, 'I get angry when I am yelled at for something I didn't do.' Avoid 'You' statements such as, 'You make me angry when you are mean.' Using I statements is a skill, just as with all communication techniques. Practice 'I' statements when you are not angry so that when you are angry, it is easier to use 'I' statements."

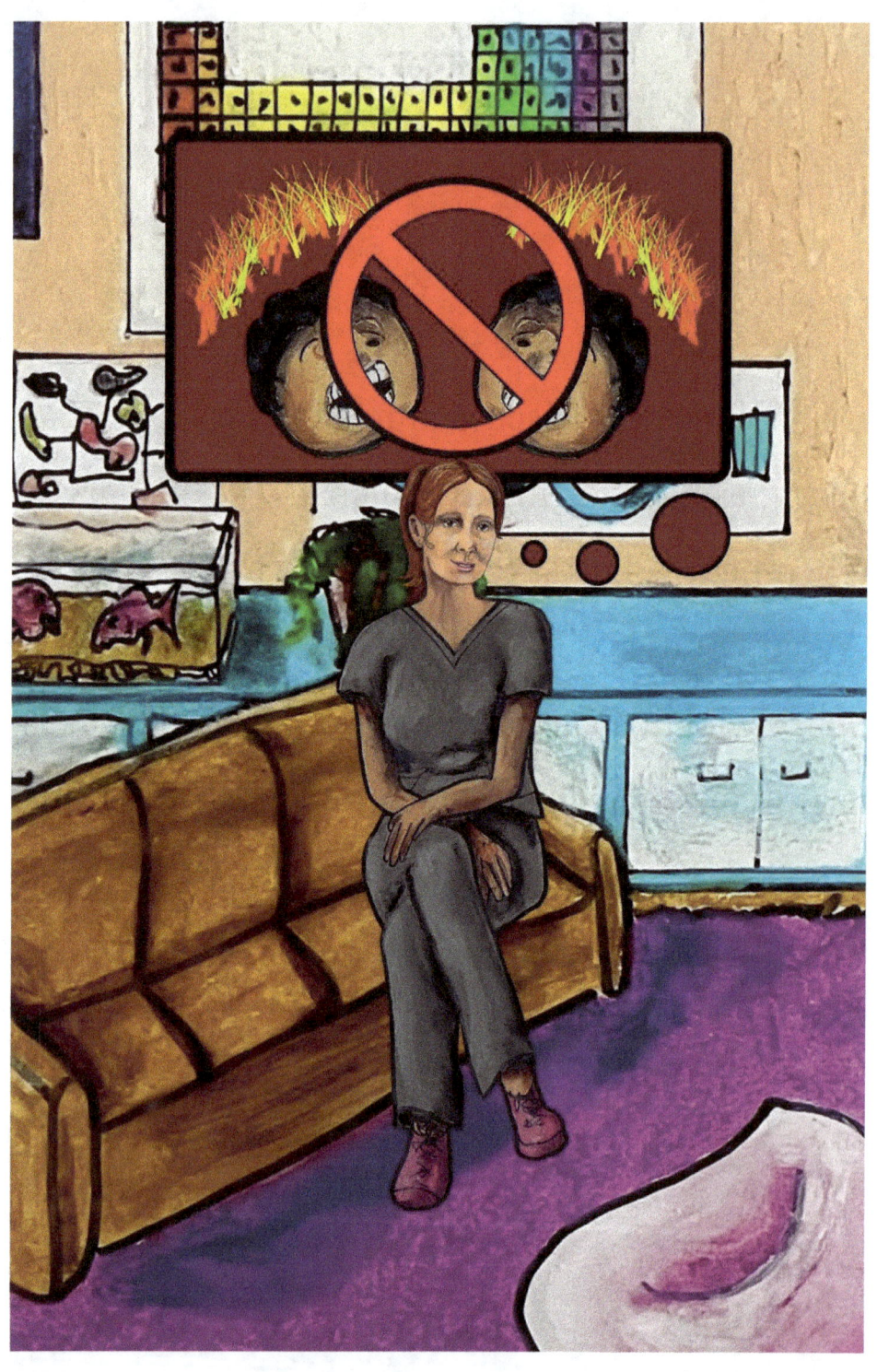

"Avoid grudges. Grudge is defined by *Merrian-Webster* as a feeling of deep-seated resentment or ill will. It is also when you are unwilling to give or admit to something. Grudges can ruin relationships. It is best to address the grudge feeling immediately with the other person, instead of holding on to it and letting it disrupt your mental equilibrium."

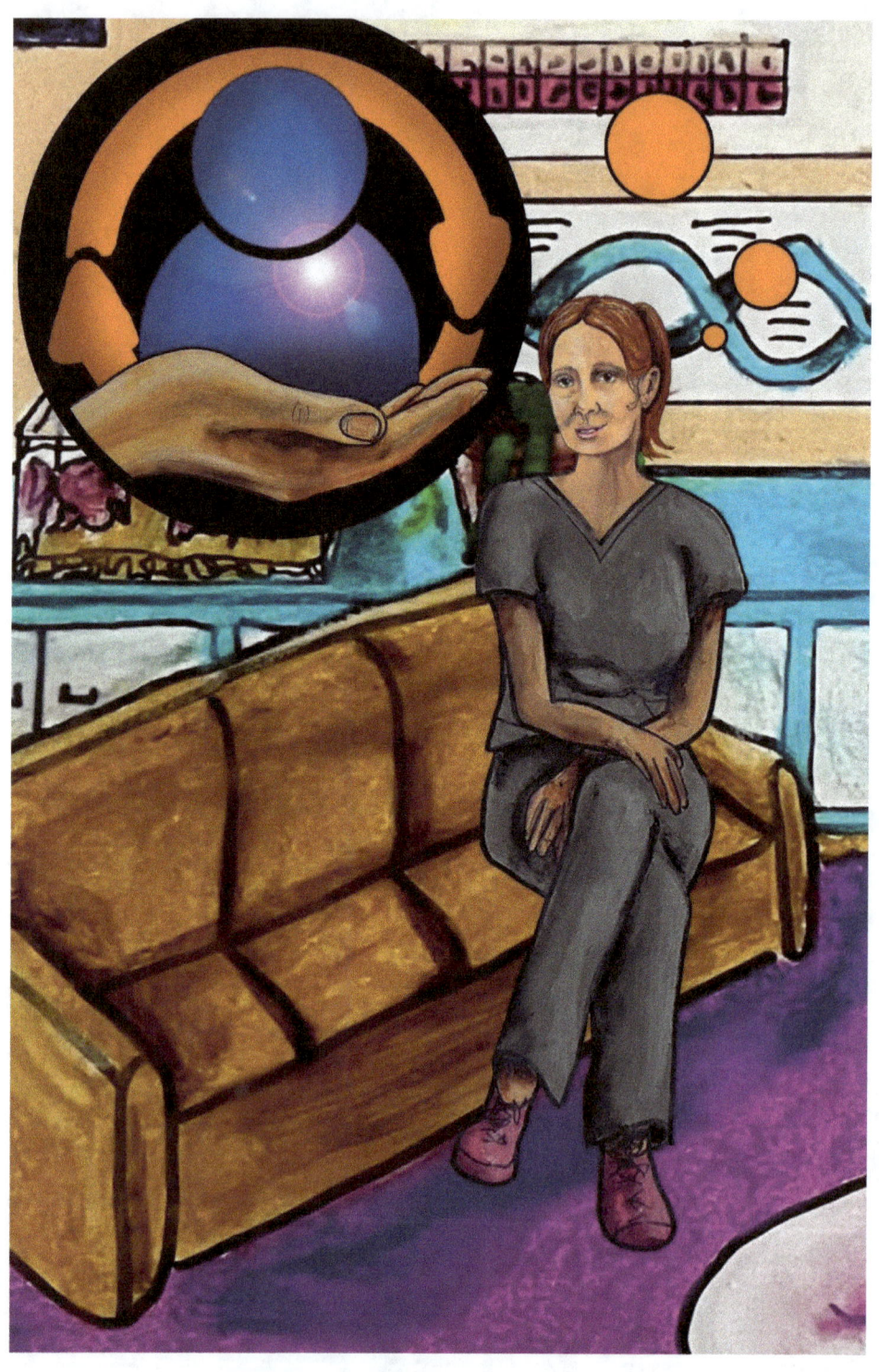

"Choose the path of adaptability and change. It is true that there are some things you may not need to change about yourself, but there are some things that you should be adaptable about. Choosing a path of adaptation can be hard sometimes, but it is worth it for a successful journey of mental well-being. Once you choose to change, do things to reinforce your decision to change, like rewarding yourself for maintaining the changed behavior."

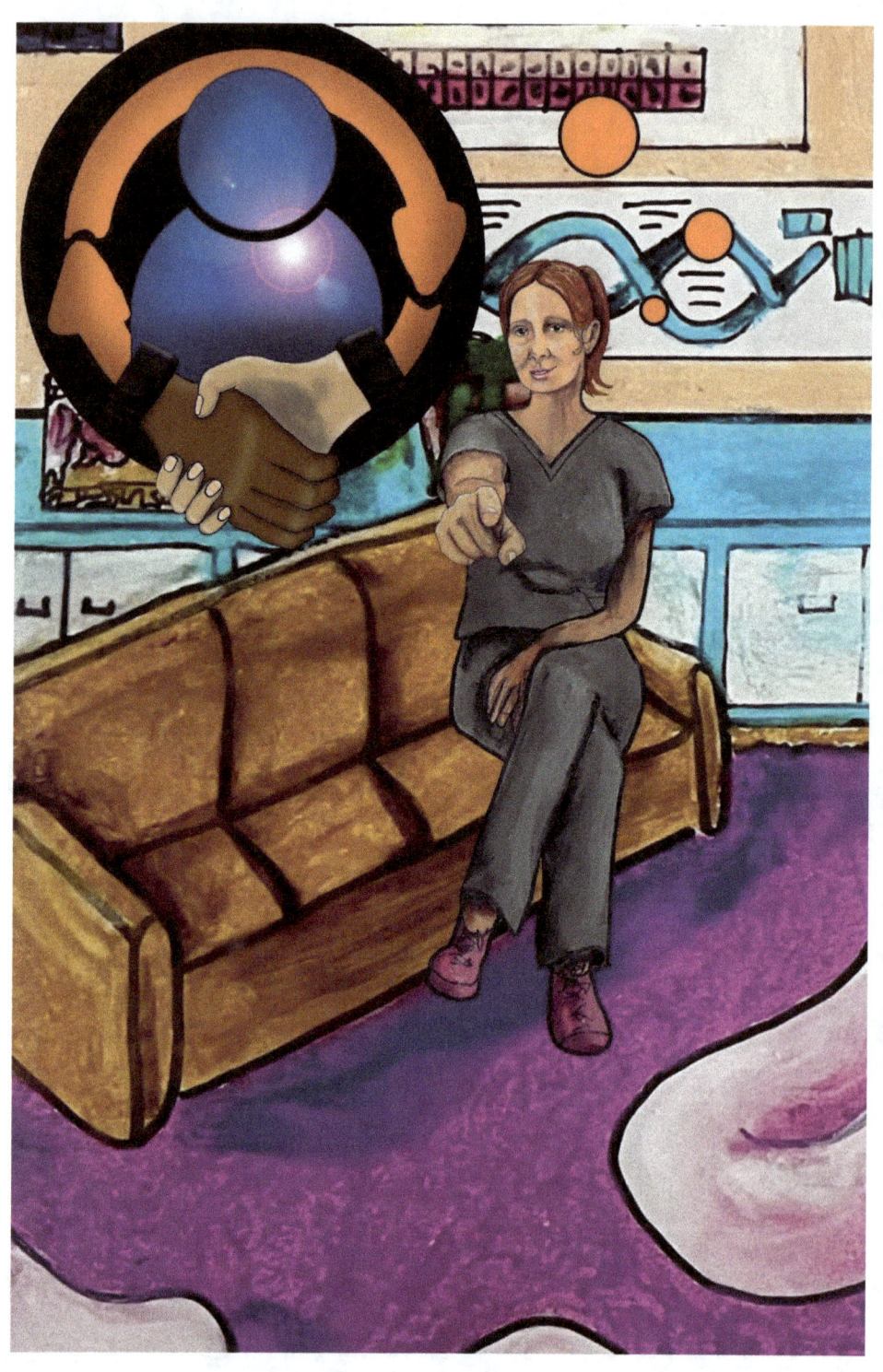

"Once you make a commitment to change and manage your anger, be vigilant and maintain high situational awareness regarding the issues or circumstances dealing with the commitment to change, so that you don't start doing old behaviors again. Commitment can be hard, and committing to change can be one of the most difficult things you can do, which is why you may need to make small incremental commitments of change. Avoid saying 'I will never do that again.' Instead, say 'I will do my best to stop myself from saying that again, and I will rehearse saying better and more appropriate things to avoid saying that again.'"

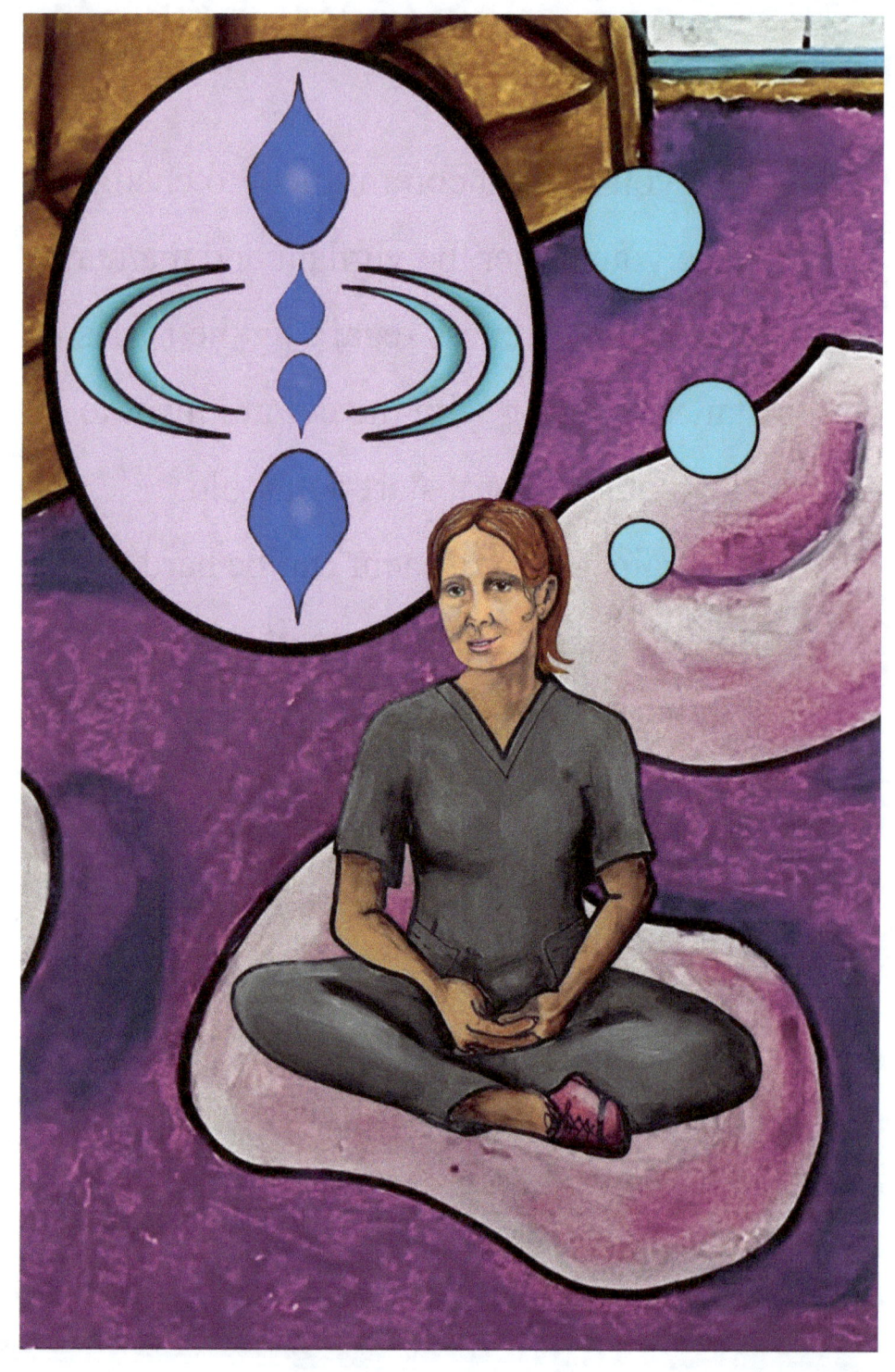

"Practicing mindfulness and being fully aware of the present moment can help you on your journey to managing anger. Practice it daily and in different situations. It is a skill worth developing."

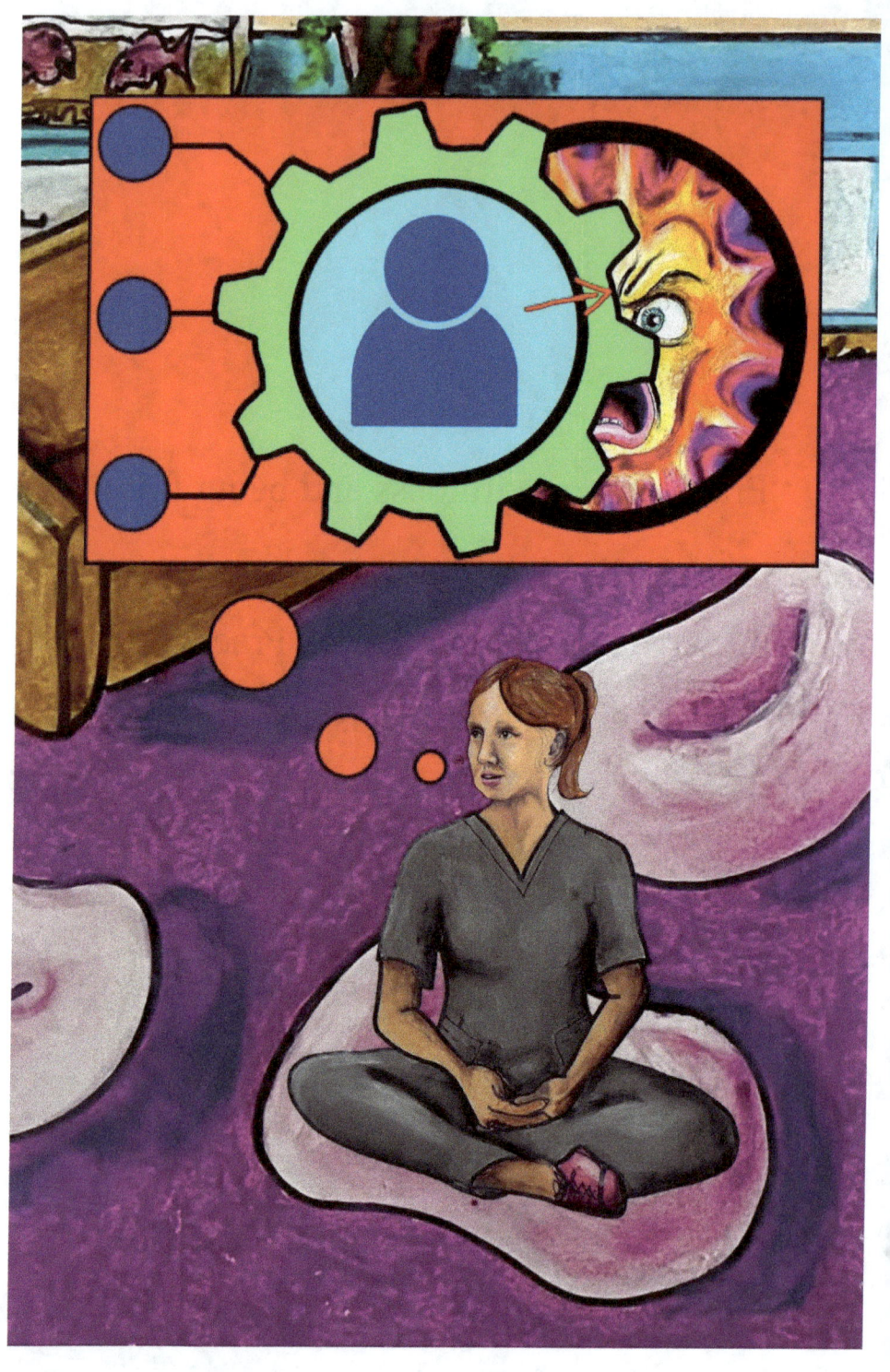

"Face your fears, and have the courage to analyze the situation with openness and honesty to see what part you may have played in causing the frustrating or irritating situation. Taking responsibility can be a first step sometimes to managing your anger."

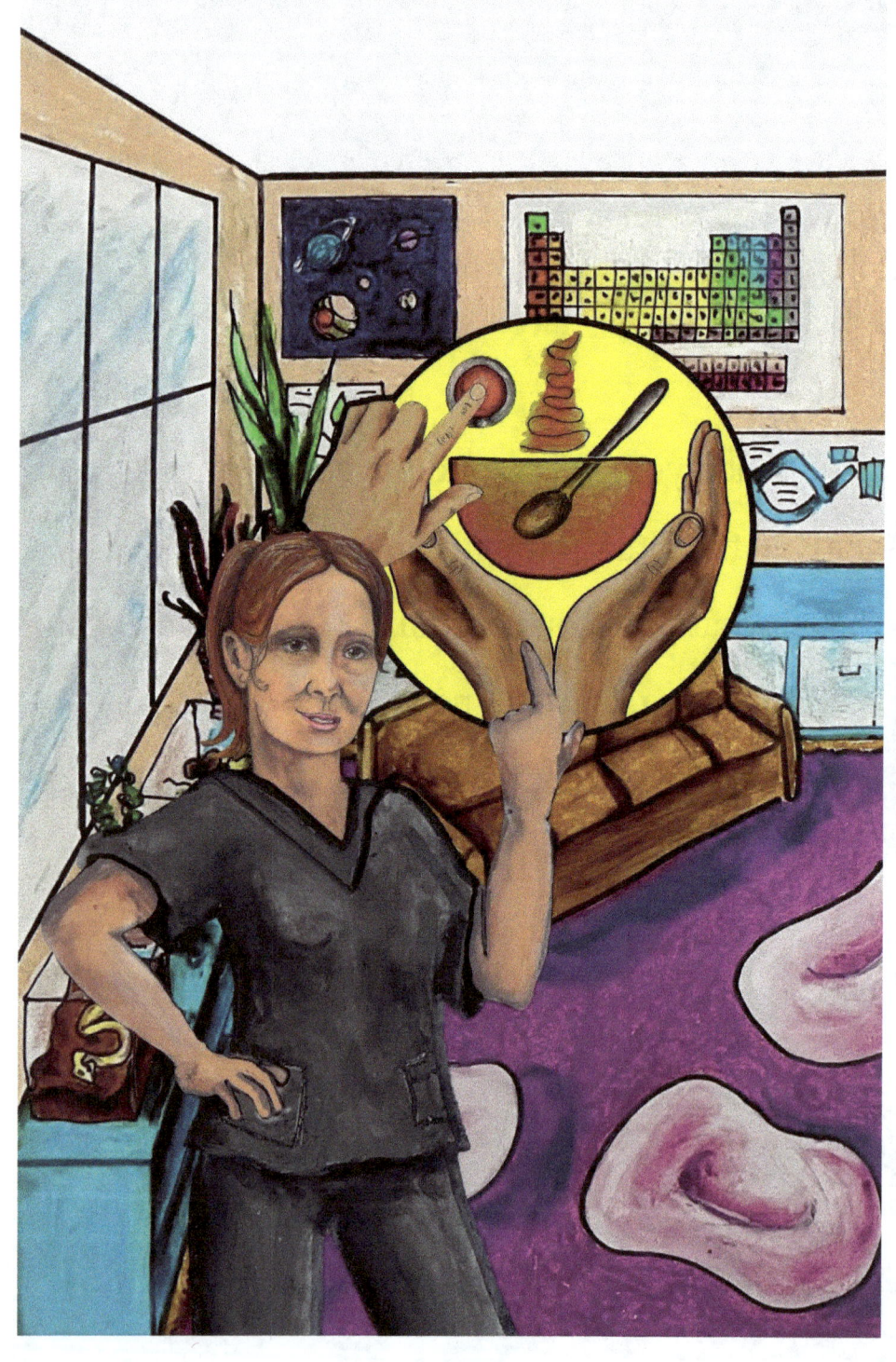

"Identify triggering states of being that may make it more likely that you become angry. Hunger can lead some people into a state of anger. Addressing your basic needs is key to avoiding recurring states of anger. Plan ahead, and keep your needs met, so that you avoid anger."

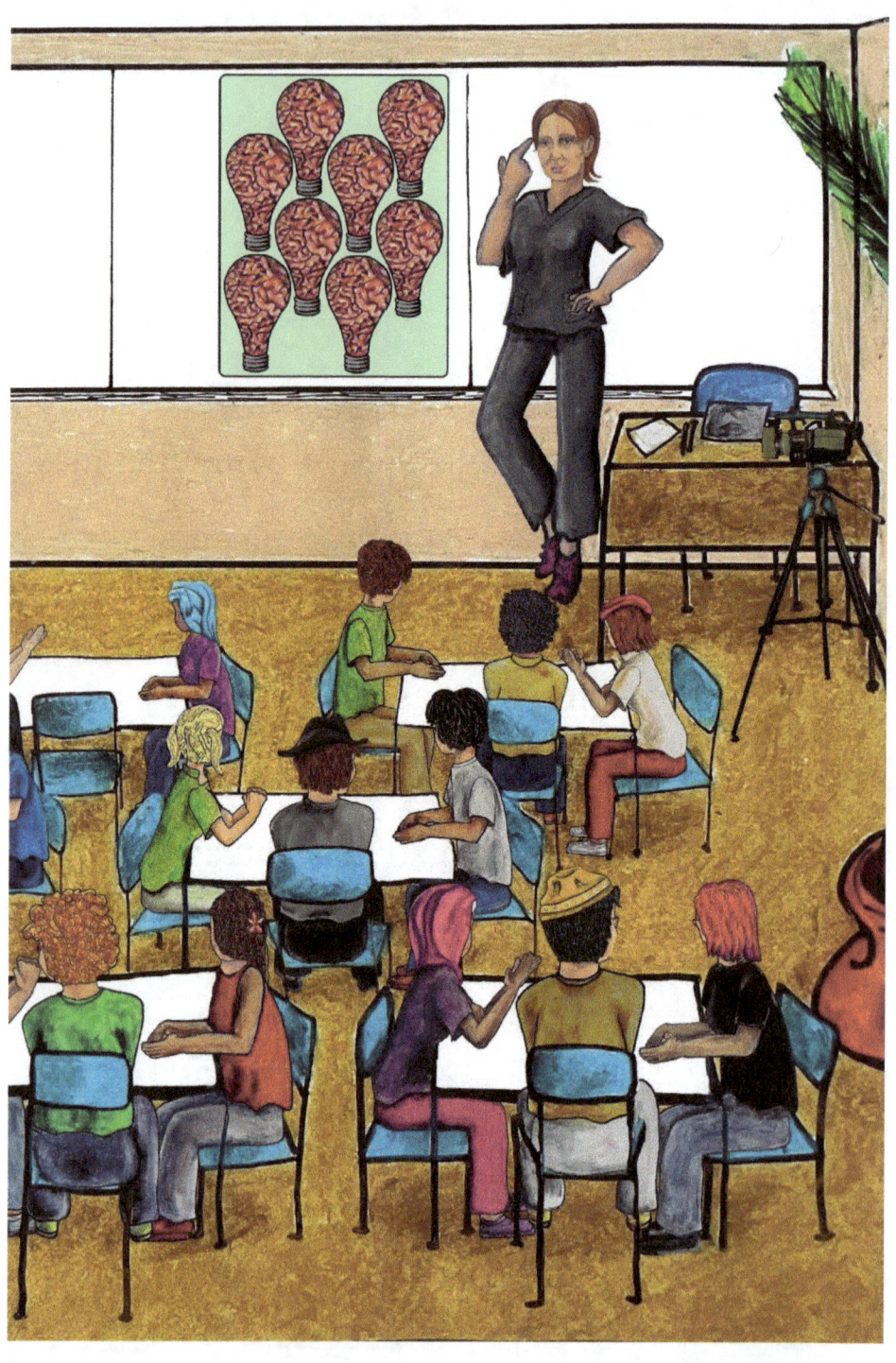

"We are unique, and we have patterns of thinking. Confront your prejudices defined by *Merriam-Webster* as an irrational attitude of hostility directed against an individual, group, race, or their supposed characteristics. Confront your bigotry, which is defined by *Merriam-Webster* as obstinate or intolerant devotion to one's own opinions and prejudices. Confront your bias, which is defined as a personal and sometimes unreasoned judgment. Confront your small-mindedness. Confront your lack of openness."

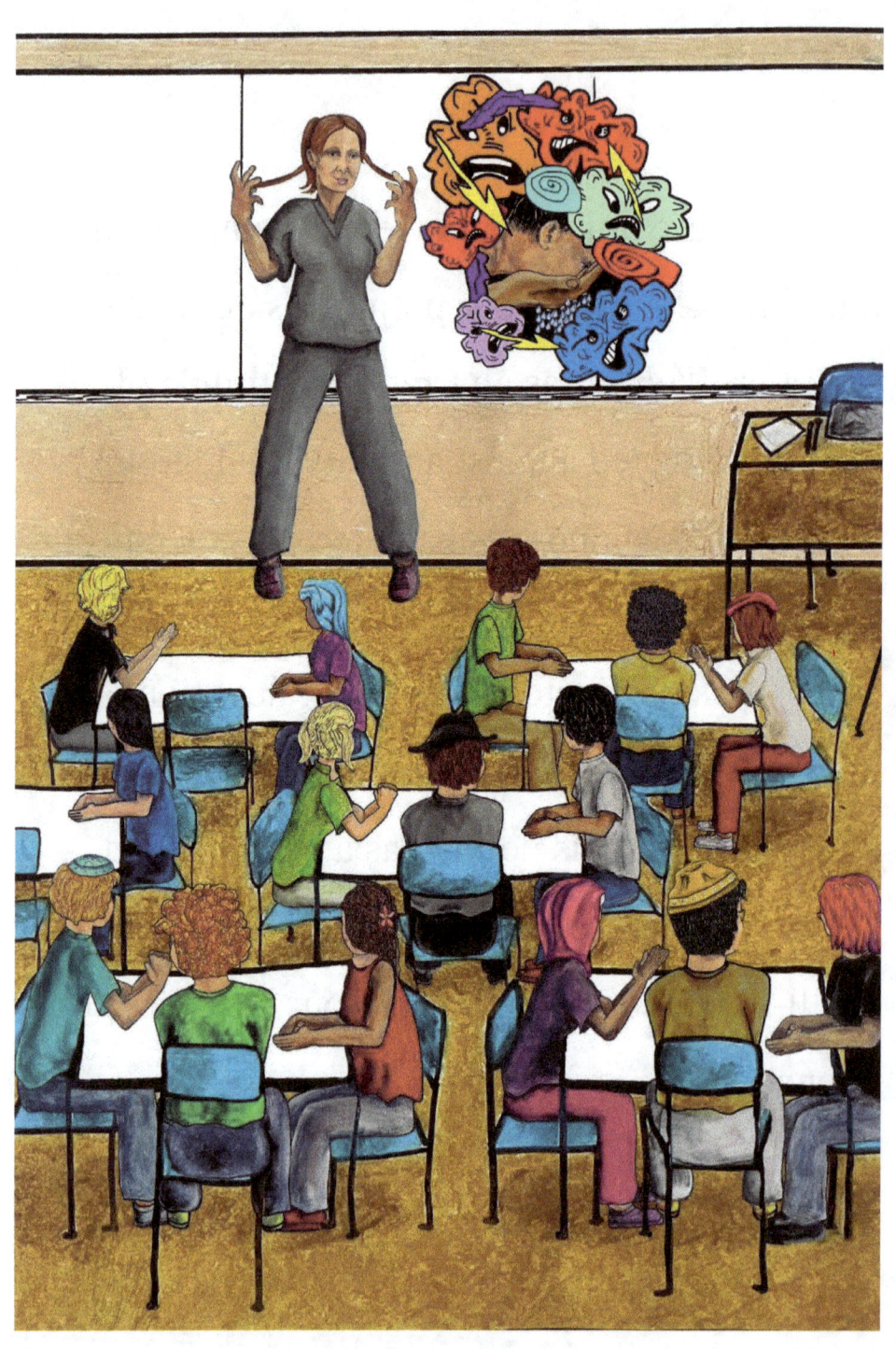

"Catastrophizing is defined by *Merriam-Webster* as imagining the worst possible outcome of an action or event, and to think about a situation or event as being a catastrophe or having a potentially catastrophic outcome. Let us not catastrophize but instead choose to see how good can come out of any situation."

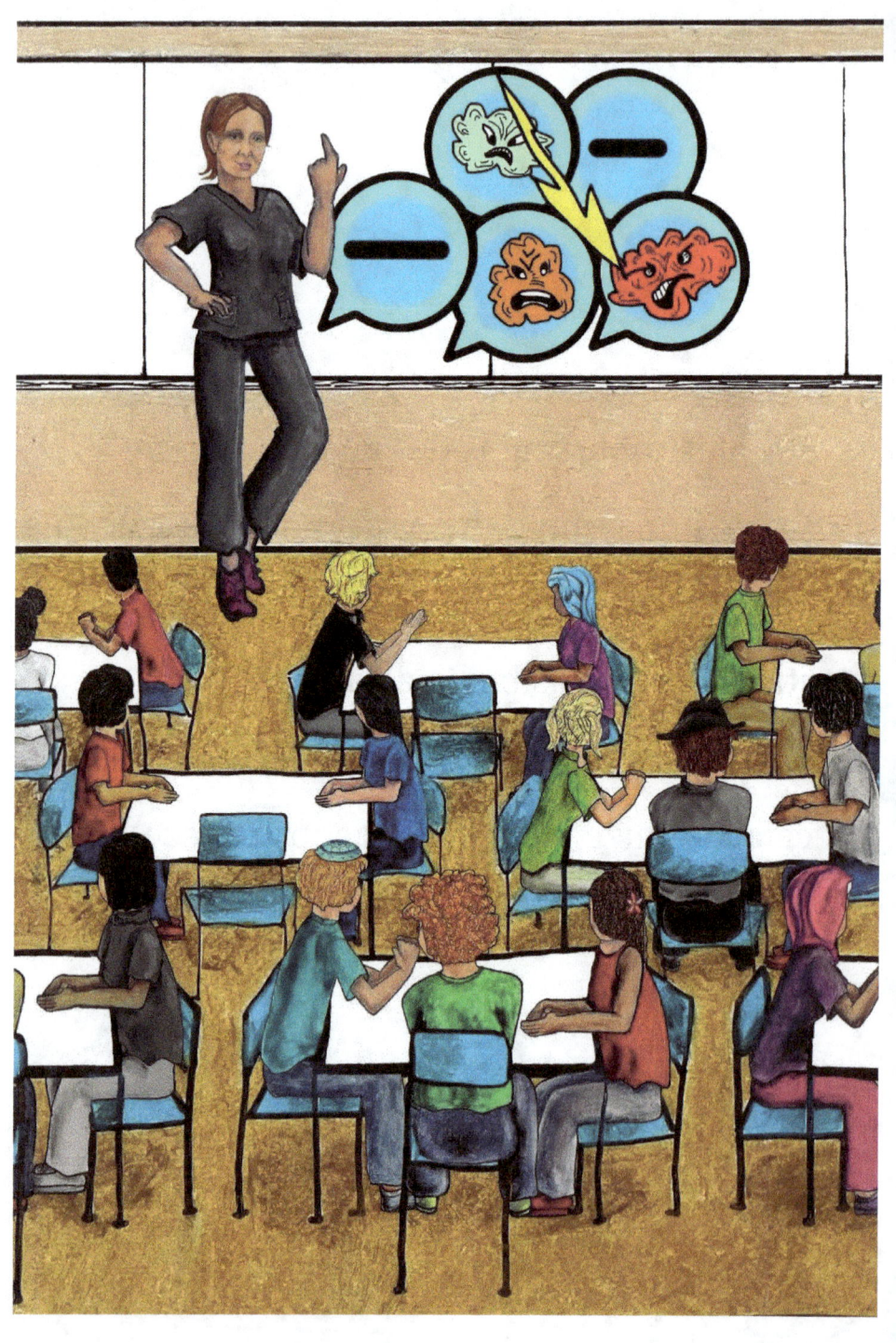

"Inflammatory labeling is also something we should avoid. This is when we give highly negative or cruel labels to people or events in our lives. This is when someone might do something you might not like, and to deal with your anger, you choose to label them in very derogatory terms like stupid, evil, and other things. Trying to understand the reason why people do things adds to the complexity that we must live in, and seeking to understand others can be better than making others try to understand us."

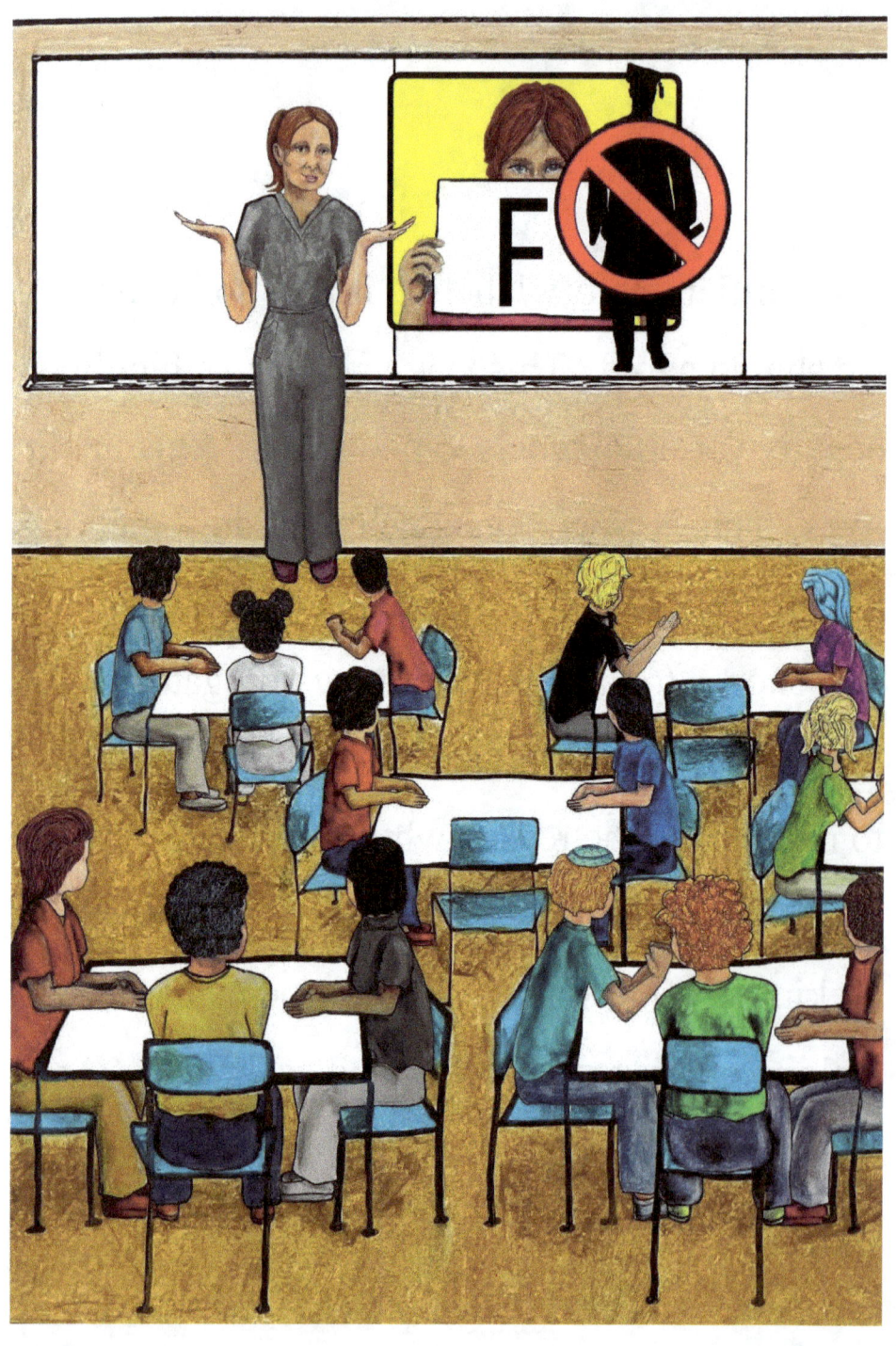

"Preventing yourself from overgeneralizing can help to manage anger. When you overgeneralize, you make broad assumptions based on limited experience, draw universal conclusions from specific events, and arrive at false conclusions based on flawed information. Basically, someone is quick to judge when they overgeneralize. Protecting your judgment from forming false conclusions is difficult, since it takes a lot of time to be patient while you gather information so that you can make an informed decision. Quick judgment can help in some circumstances but should not be viewed as a skill that needs to be developed in every situation and event. Making broad assumptions about many things is something that young people do, but we need to mature and grow in our abilities to withhold judgment until information is received."

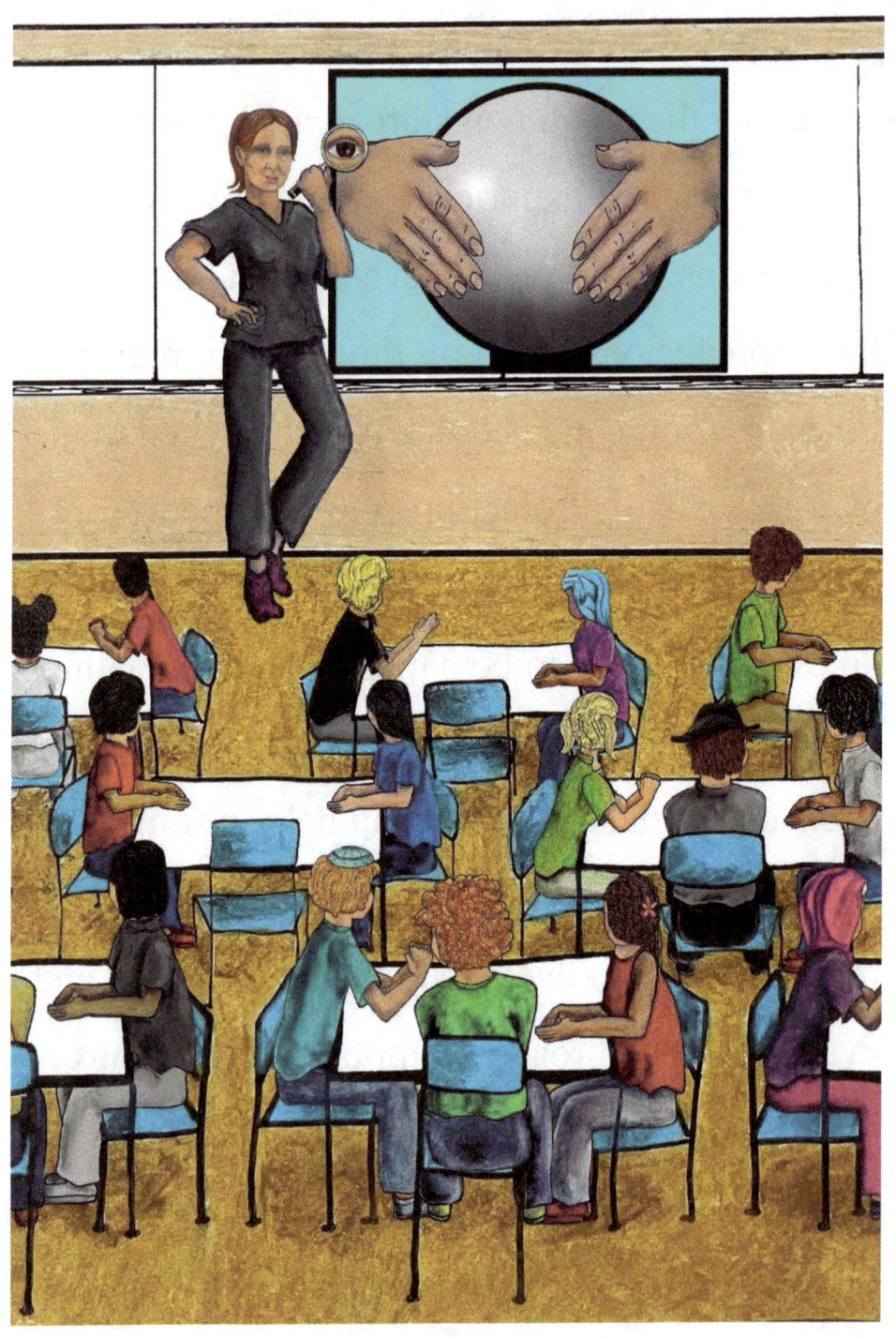

"Thinking you can predict the future correctly all the time can be seen as fortune telling. This should be avoided since the world is so complex and events unfold in unpredictable ways many times. Be a good observer, watch things, and adapt to them. Trying to predict the future and believing you are always right can lead to frustration and anger since it is unpredictable."

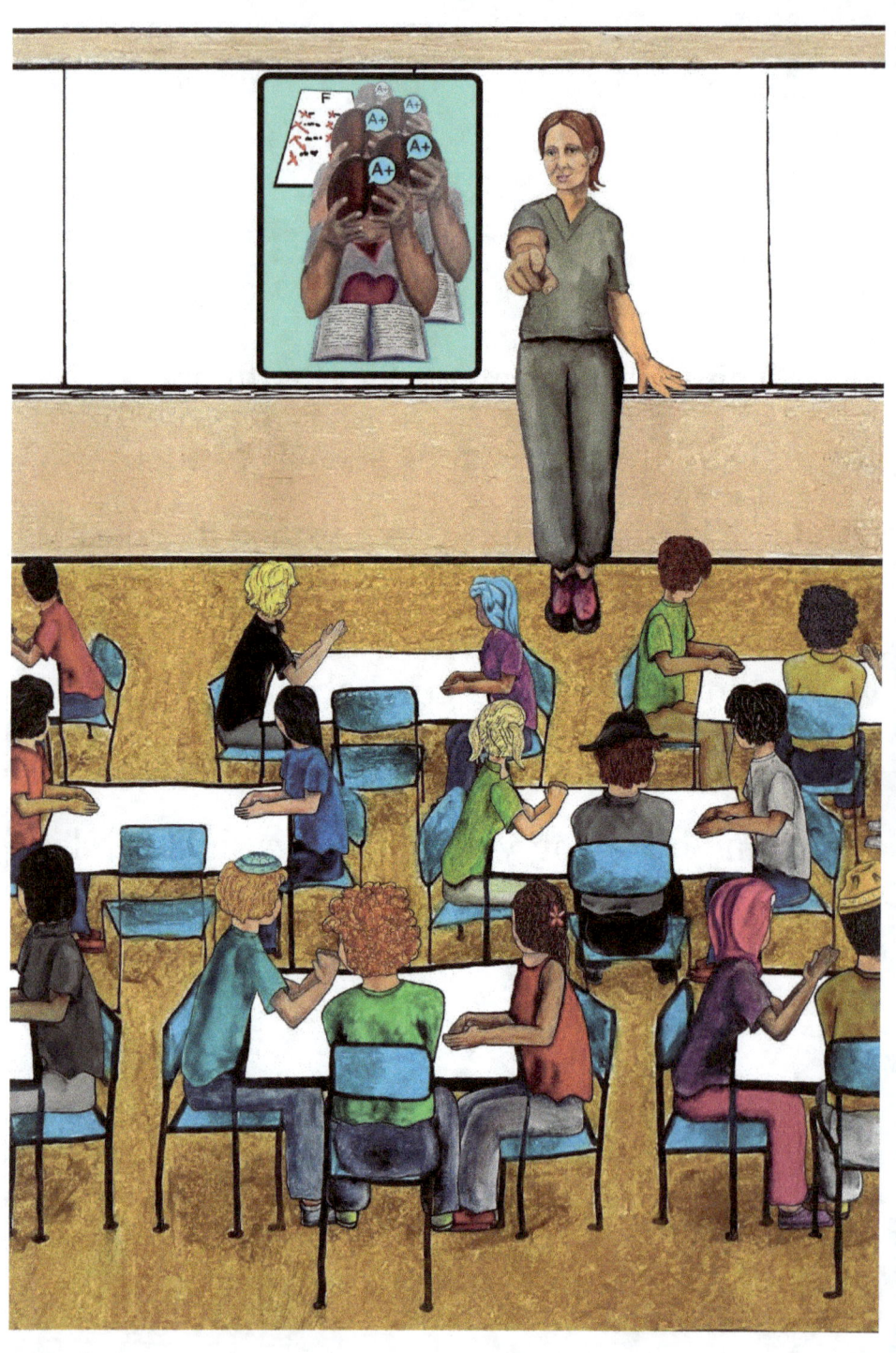

"Do things to increase your self-efficacy or belief in your capabilities. Try new hobbies and learn new things every year. Try learning a new language. Increase your skillset for the sake of learning and growth. This will help increase your self-confidence and help you be more resilient when you face situations that could make you angry, since it may be hard to see how to resolve the problem. Increasing your skills will better prepare you to face the unknown future."

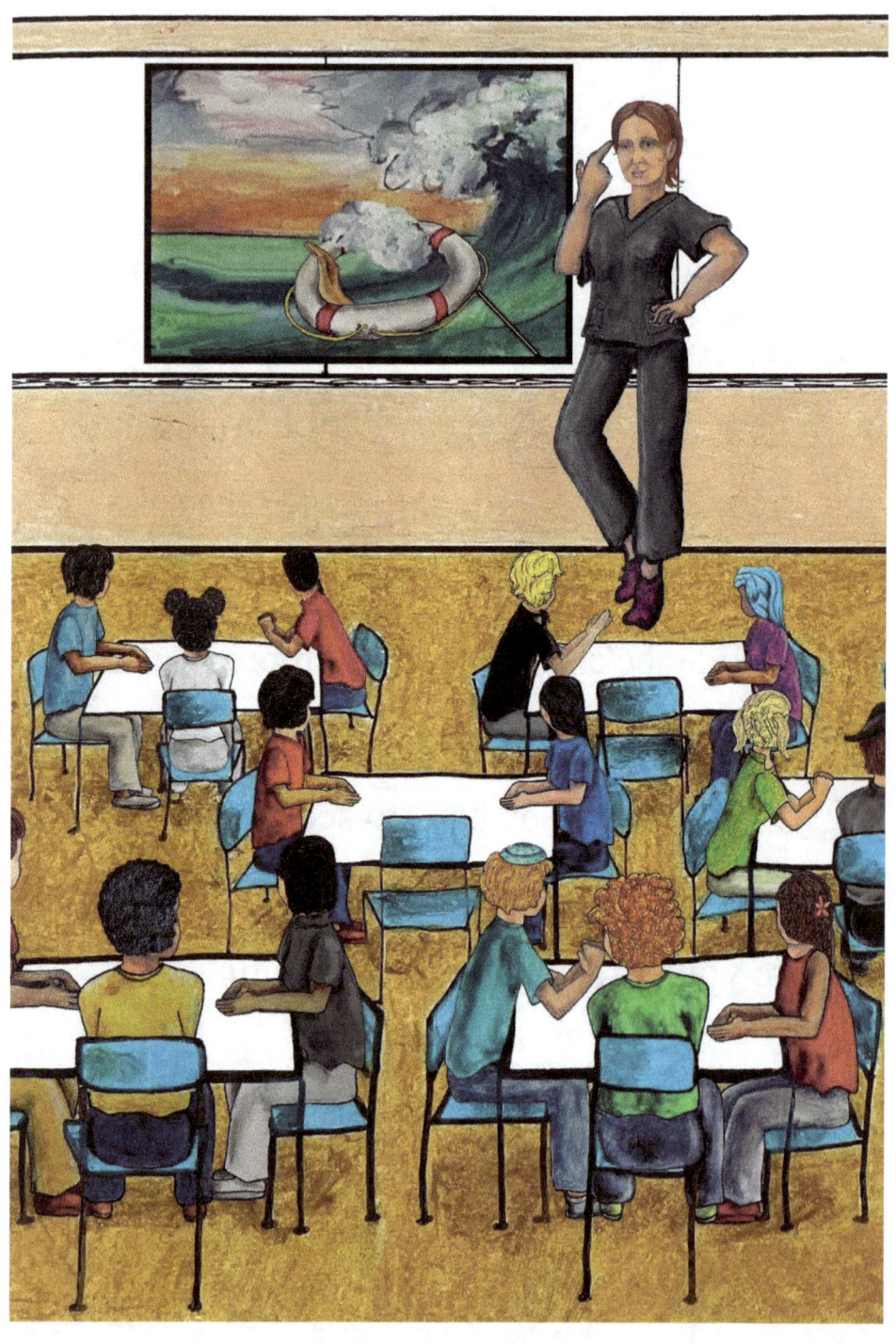

"Develop crisis survival skills when faced with anger. An easy step may be to just leave the situation. Learn to distract yourself so that you can try to view the situation as it is and how it can be resolved. Create strong sensations like listening to music that is elevated in volume but not harmful to the inner ear. Eat peppermint or very sour candy. Smell lavender oil. Learn to release your energy related to anger through healthy ways like creating art, journaling, or creating music."

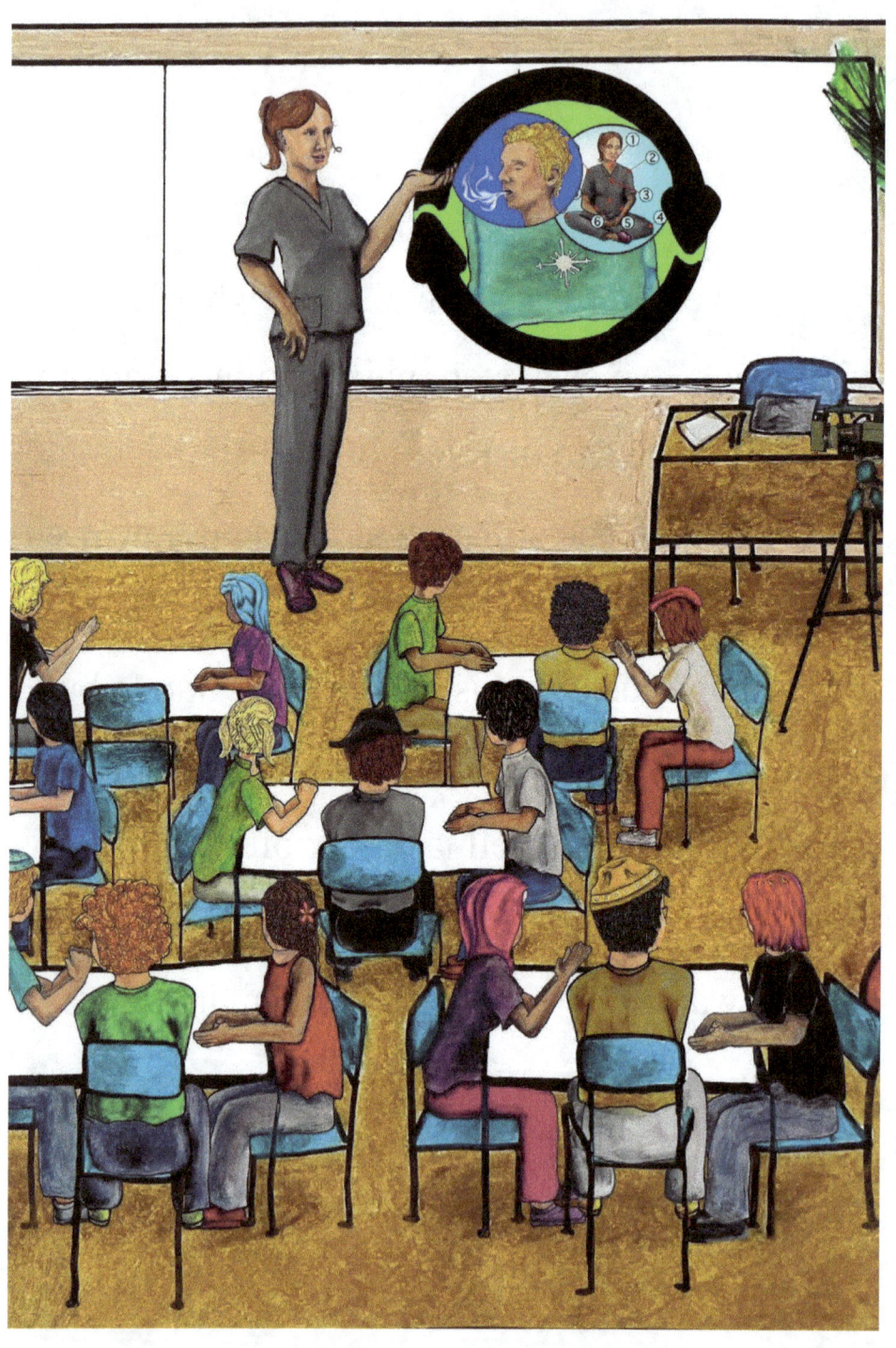

"You can do things such as changing your physical sensations. This could include changing your breathing through deep breathing. You can do progressive muscle relaxation to relax all your muscles. You can lower your body temperature if you have some ice available. Changing your bodily sensations can distract you from your anger."

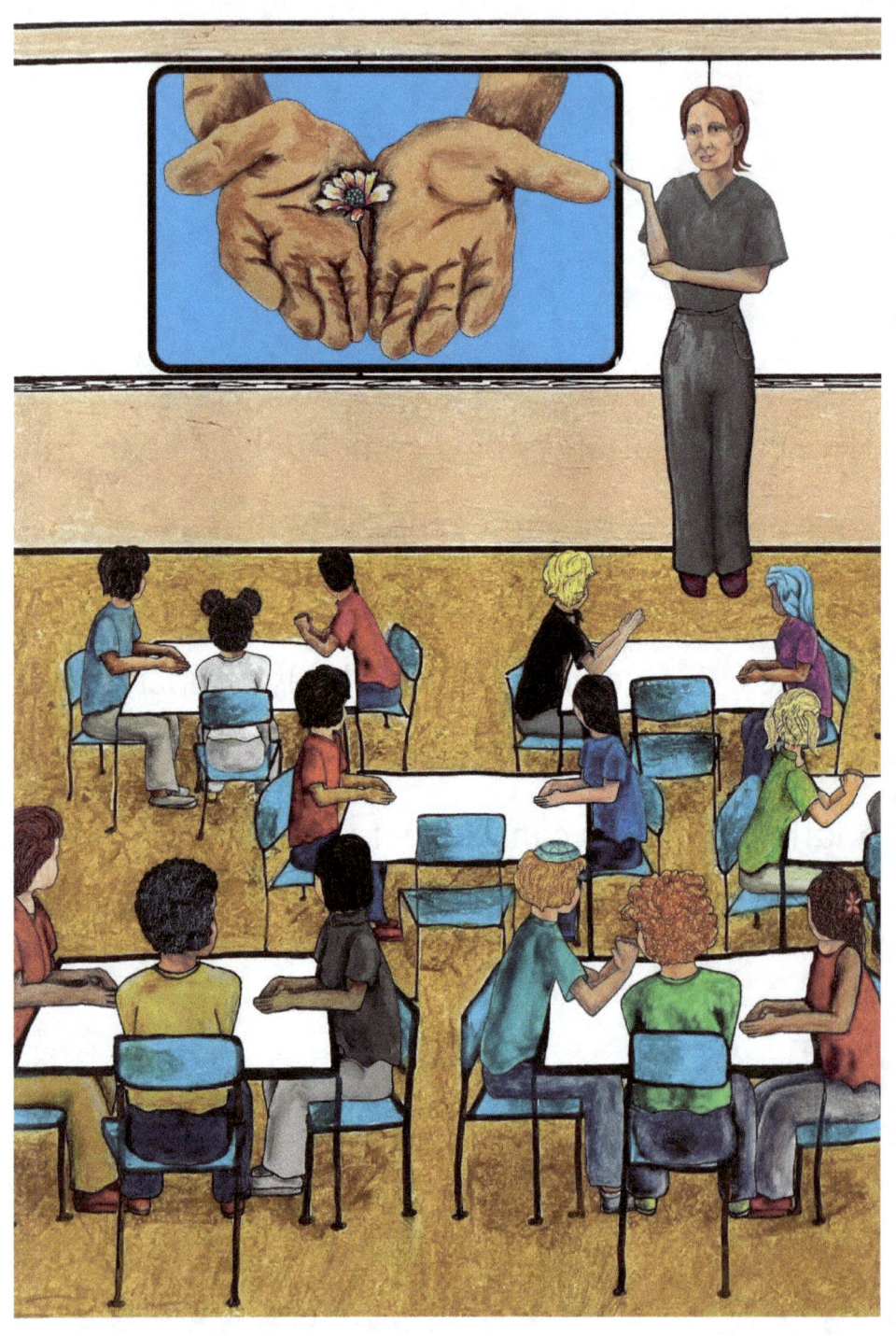

"Develop reality acceptance skills. This can simply start by doing the 5 senses exercise, where you notice things in the room you are in with all your senses, such as noticing things that are blue in the room, listening to what you hear in the room, feeling the clothes on your body, and other things. Accepting what is real can help you sometimes with anger management by recognizing your situation as it is, and realizing that it is there for different reasons. Once you accept reality as it is, it will be easier to come up with a plan to change the things you can change. It takes wisdom to know what the things in life are that you can change and which things you must accept as they are without changing them. Ask the Universe for wisdom to know which things you should and must change."

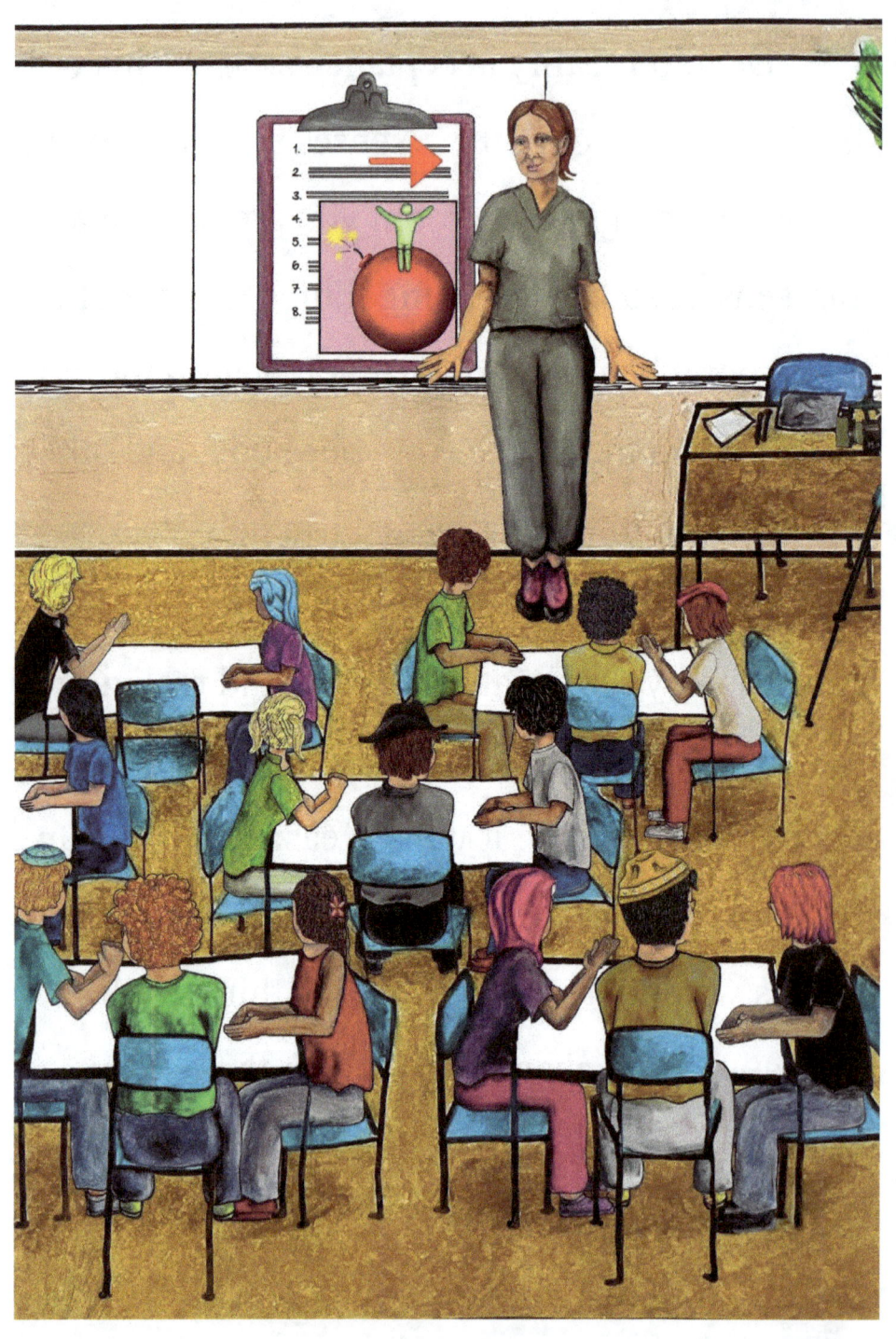

"We will all face difficult situations at some point, so it is best to start planning for them. Make a list of things you need to be prepared for. Develop goals on how to acquire the things you need. Prepare plans to use the resources you will have for your future event, so that frustration and anxiety will be minimized when the time comes to put your plan into action."

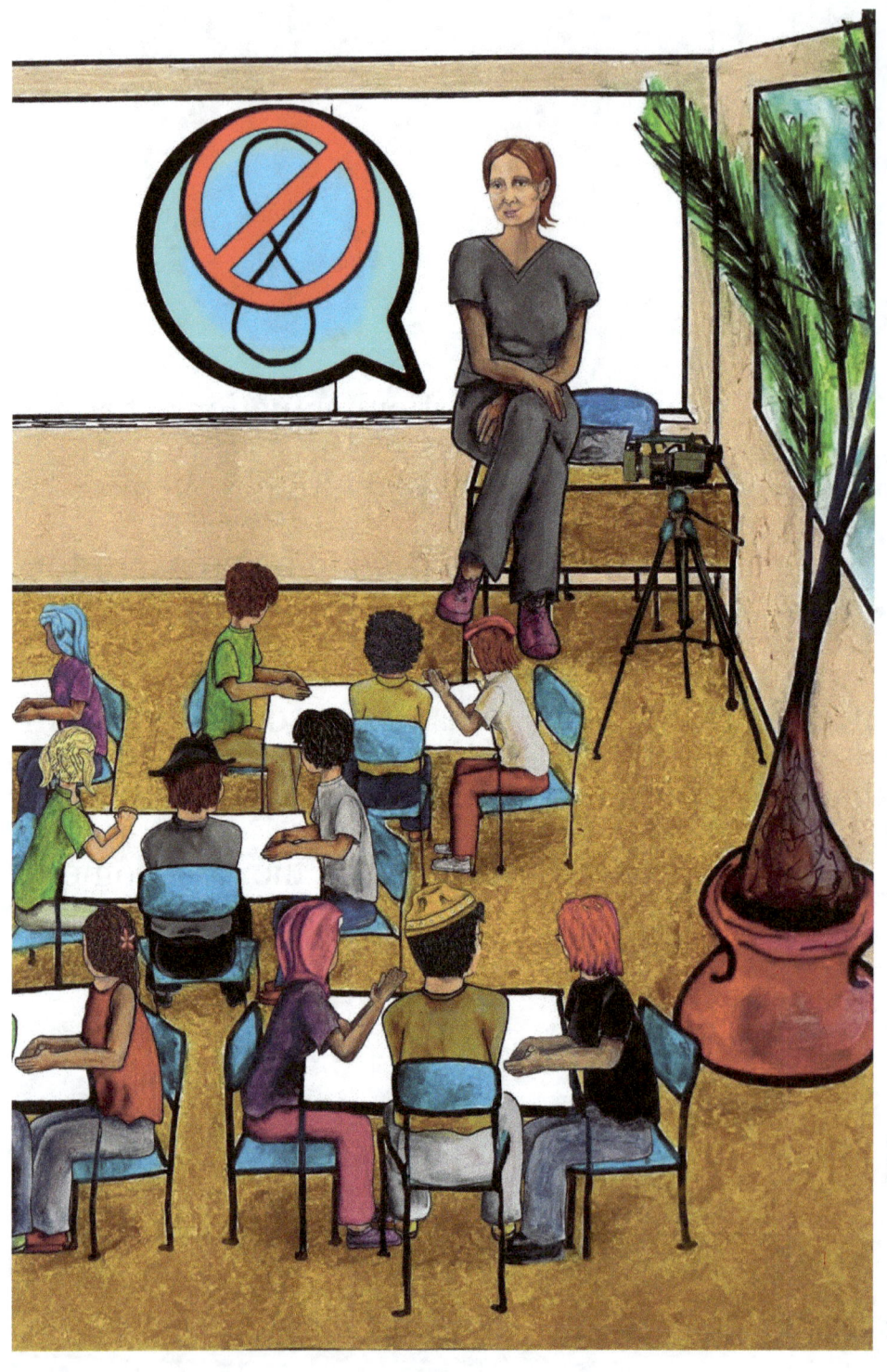

"Avoid using the words never and always. Few things in life are never going to happen or will always happen."

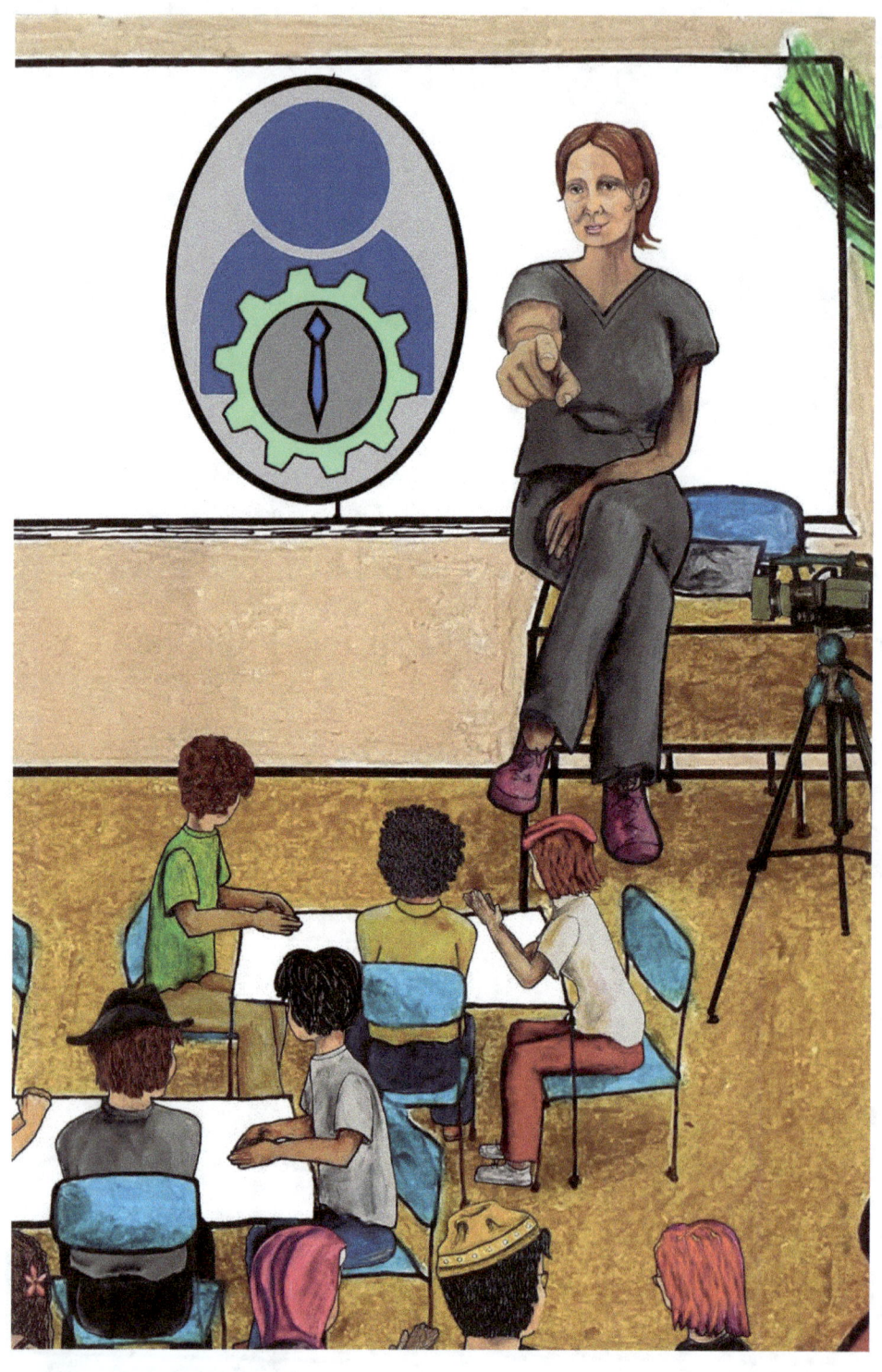

"Become a professional in whatever career you choose. Professionalism in one area of life can easily be applied to other areas of life. Being a professional can help you stay organized and manage things. Learning to manage one thing very well can help you manage anger."

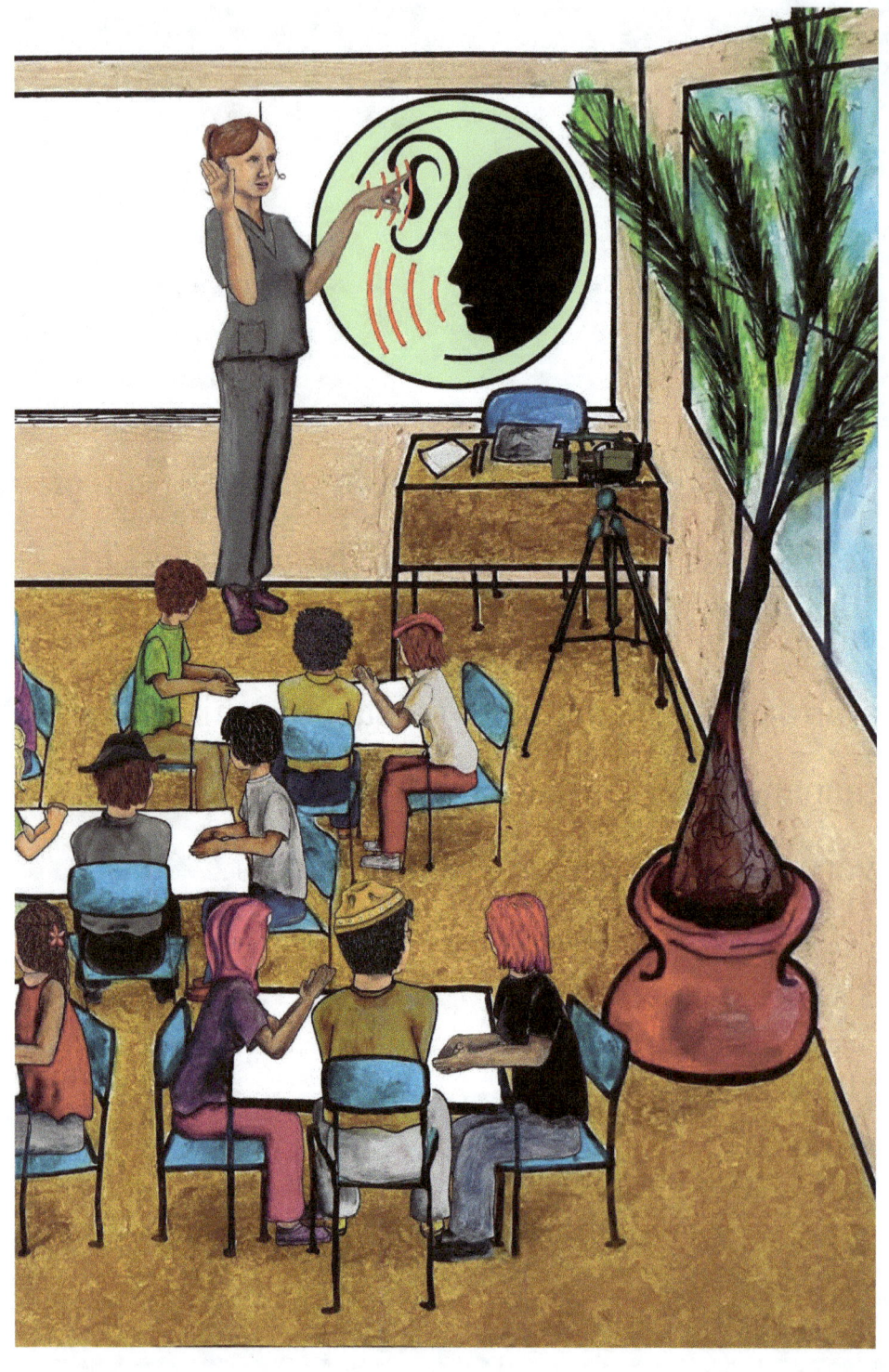

"When you are in a verbal argument, learn to try to listen to the other person instead of just stopping to talk until it is your turn to say whatever it is you wanted to say. Conversations evolve, and something you may have wanted to say at the beginning of an argument may not be applicable anymore toward the end of the argument."

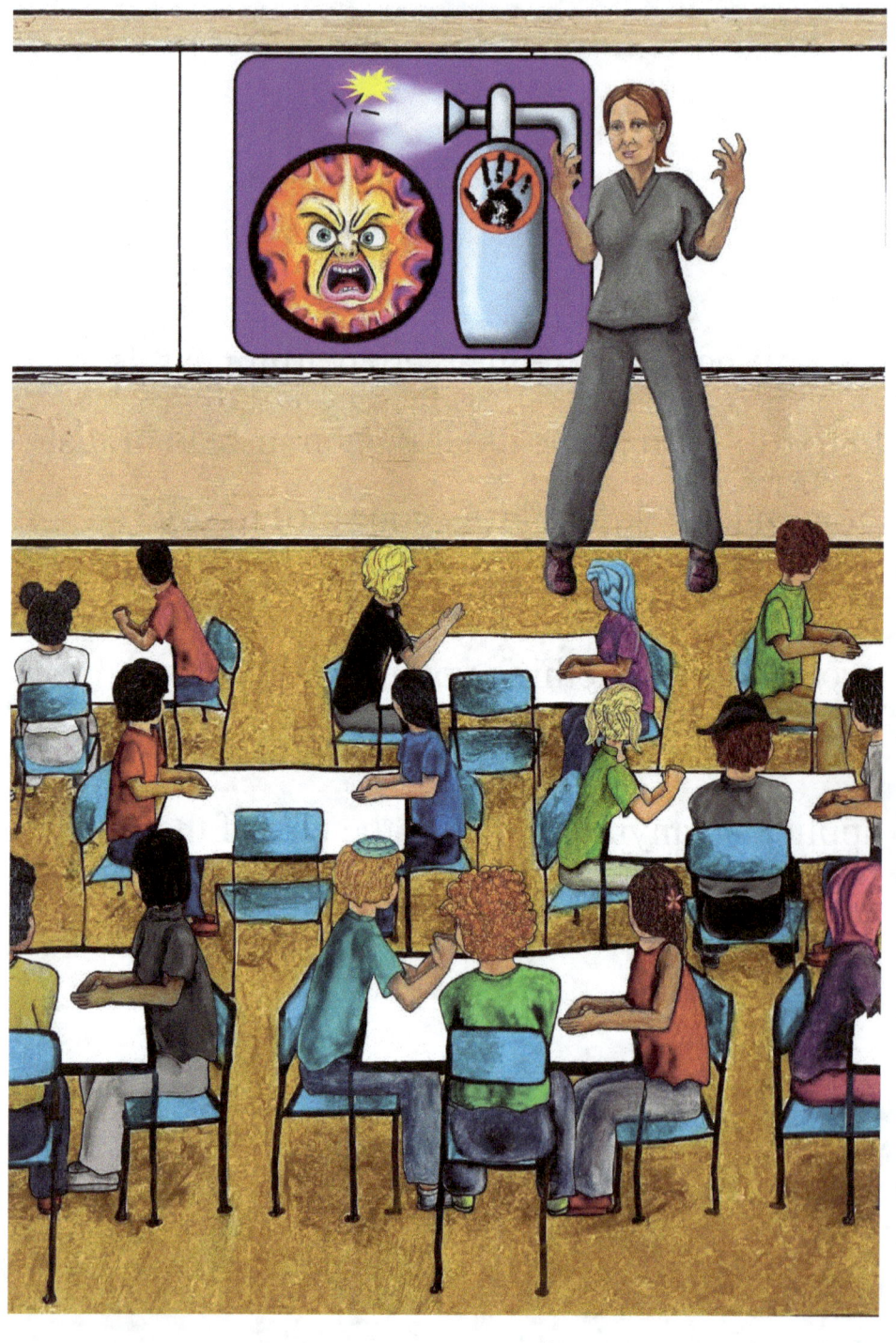

"Avoid suppressing your anger. It is ok to leave the situation or stay silent so that you don't do something you will regret, but avoid suppressing the emotion of anger so that it never comes out of you. Anger is a natural emotion and must be properly dealt with."

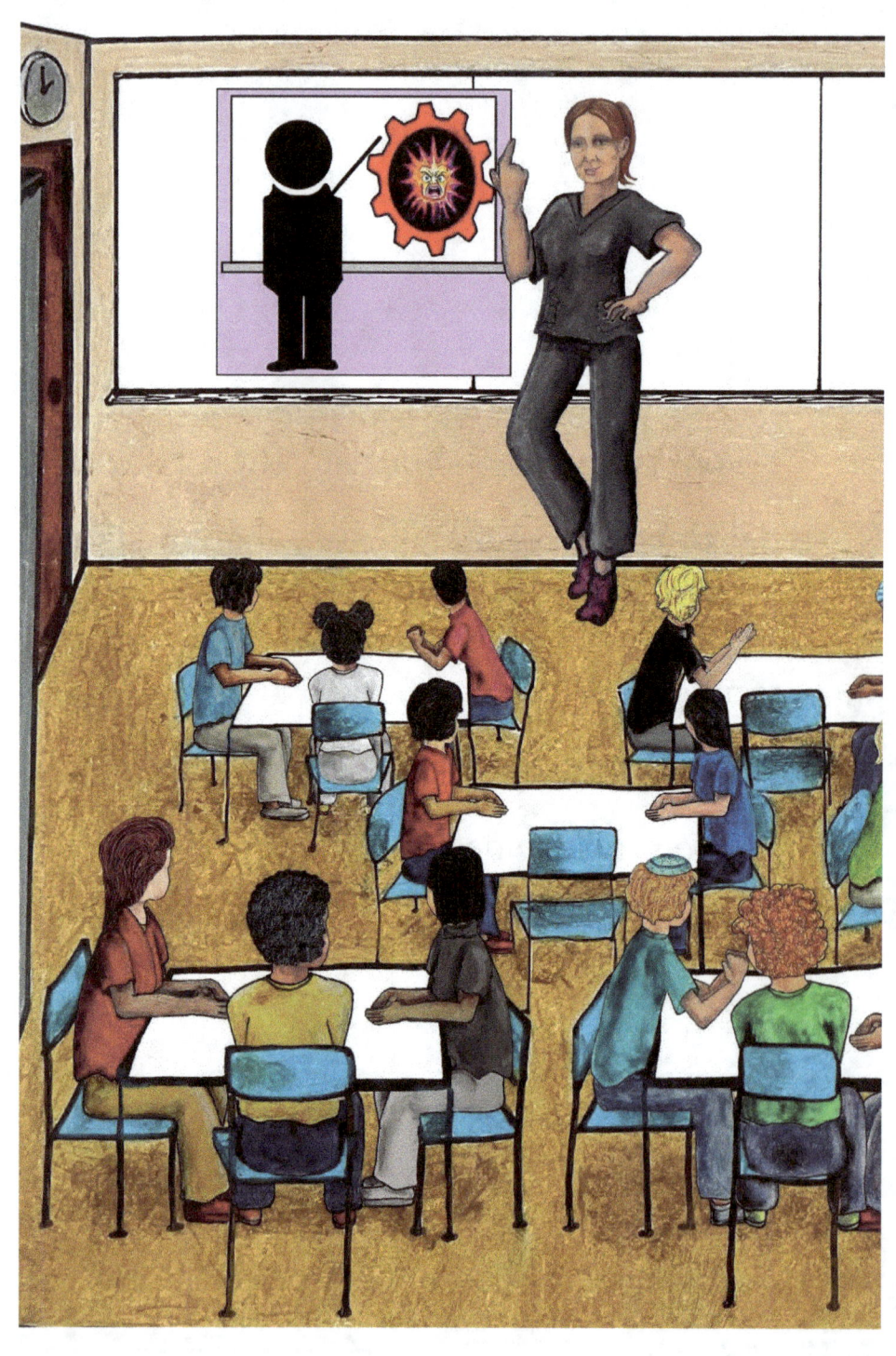

"Some people may need to attend an anger management class or workshop, so that they gain more skills to manage their anger. Ask a social worker about available classes in your area or online."

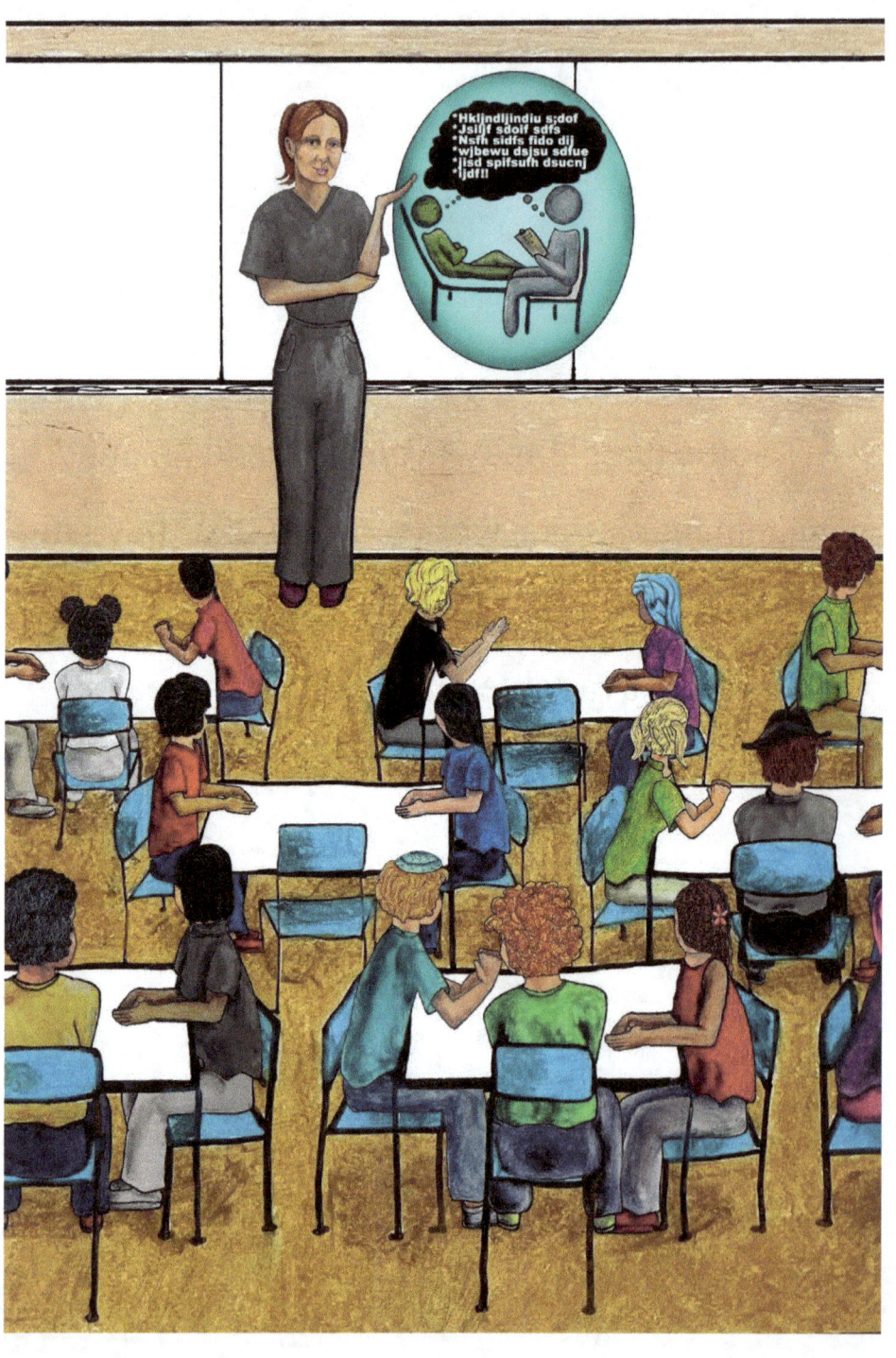

"Some people may need to see a therapist to manage their anger. Talking to someone with a lot of experience helping others deal with their emotions can be very beneficial. Therapy takes courage to start and to finish."

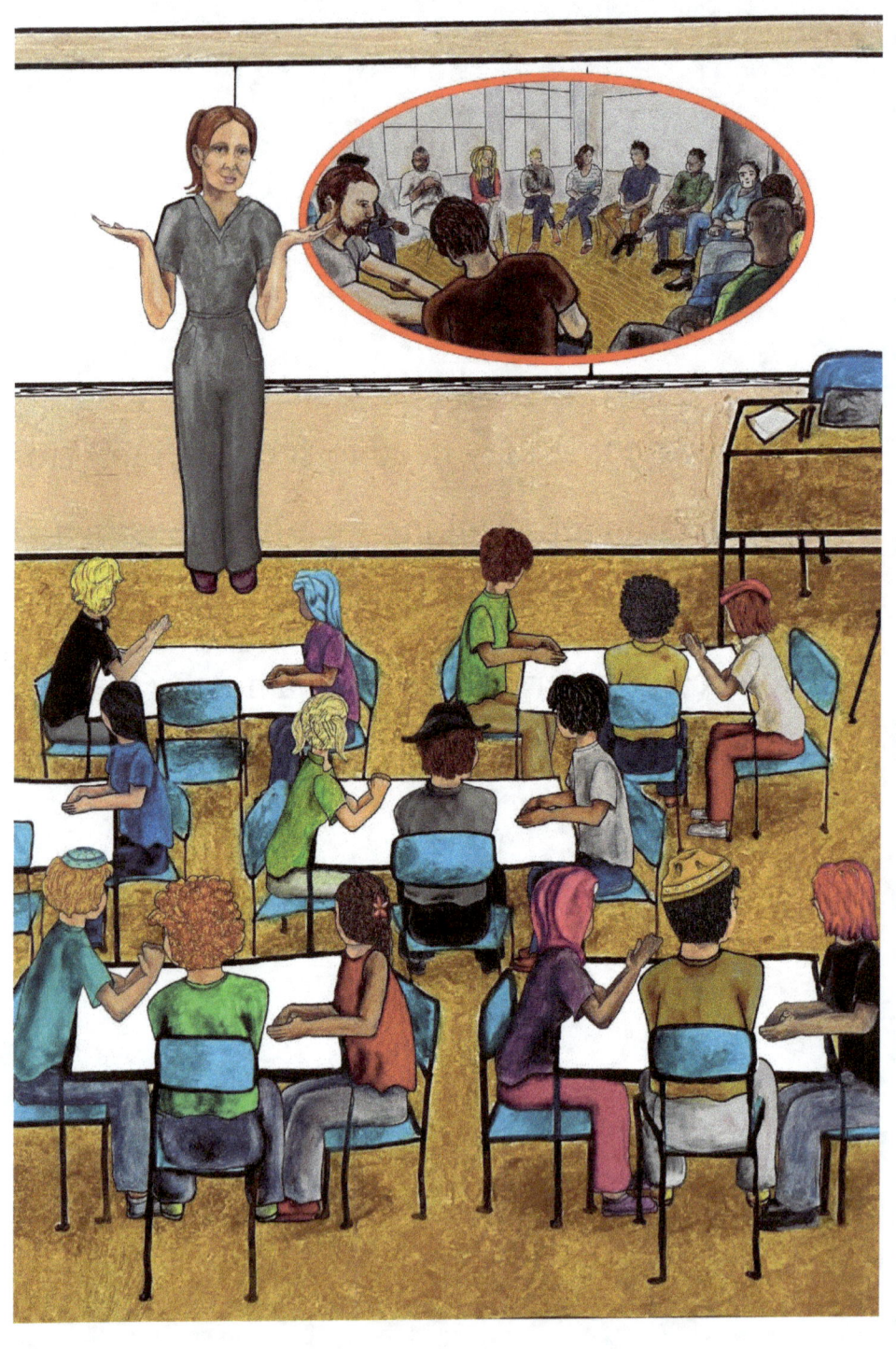

"Some people may benefit from group therapy, where everyone dealing with a similar experience processes their feelings as a group. This also takes courage since you will have to open up and talk to strangers about your raw feelings. We were all strangers at some point, though."

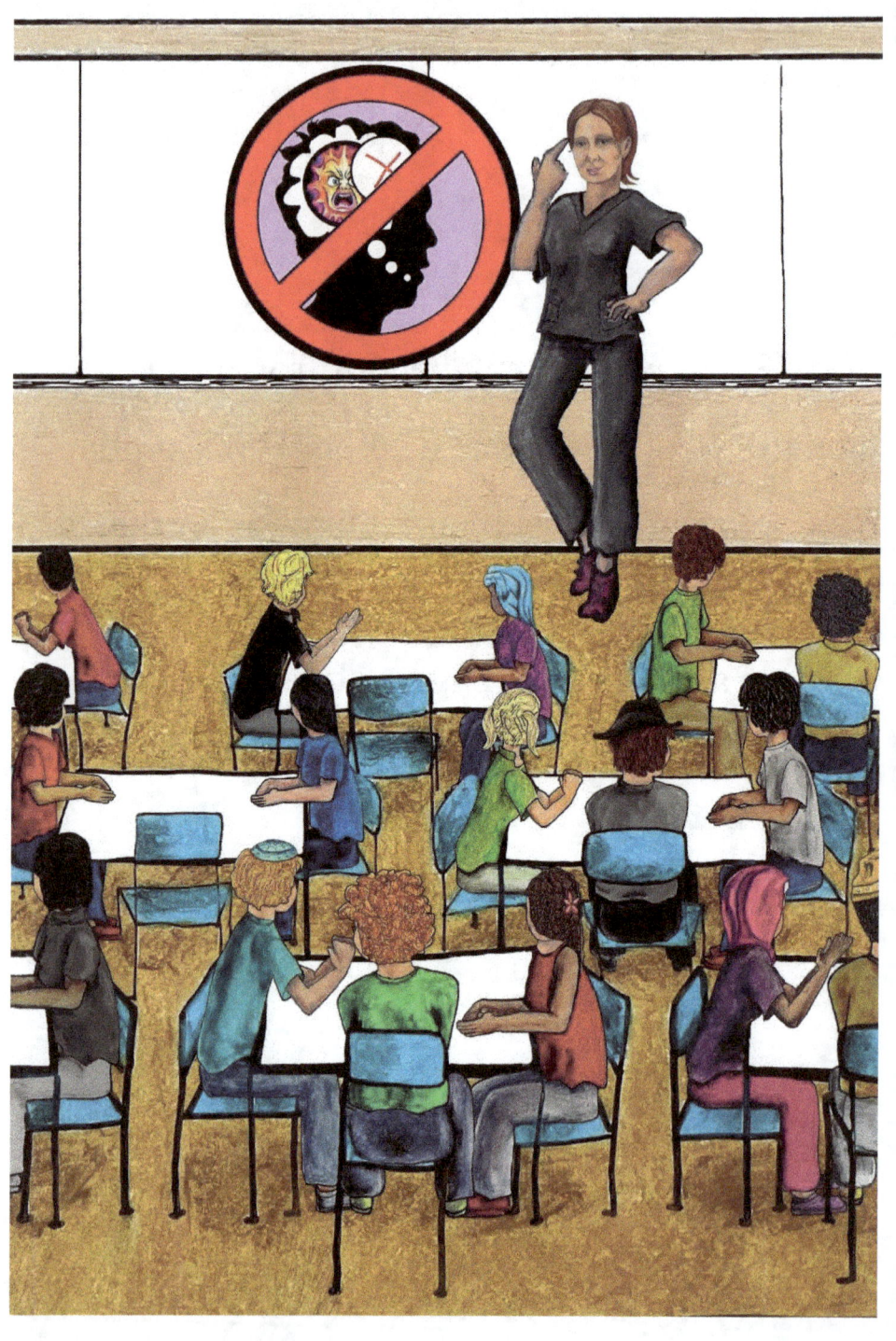

"When you deal with other people's anger, avoid dismissing their anger just to try to get them to stop being angry. Everyone's experience is unique and valid, so we must try to understand others and help them on their journey. Try not to deflect a person's anger onto someone else who does not deserve it or is not responsible for it. Help the other person carefully observe their situation so that they place their anger toward the correct person, thing, or situation. Don't automatically defend someone for being angry before you know why they are angry. You should be willing to confront someone who is angry and help them realize that their anger is misplaced when it is misplaced."

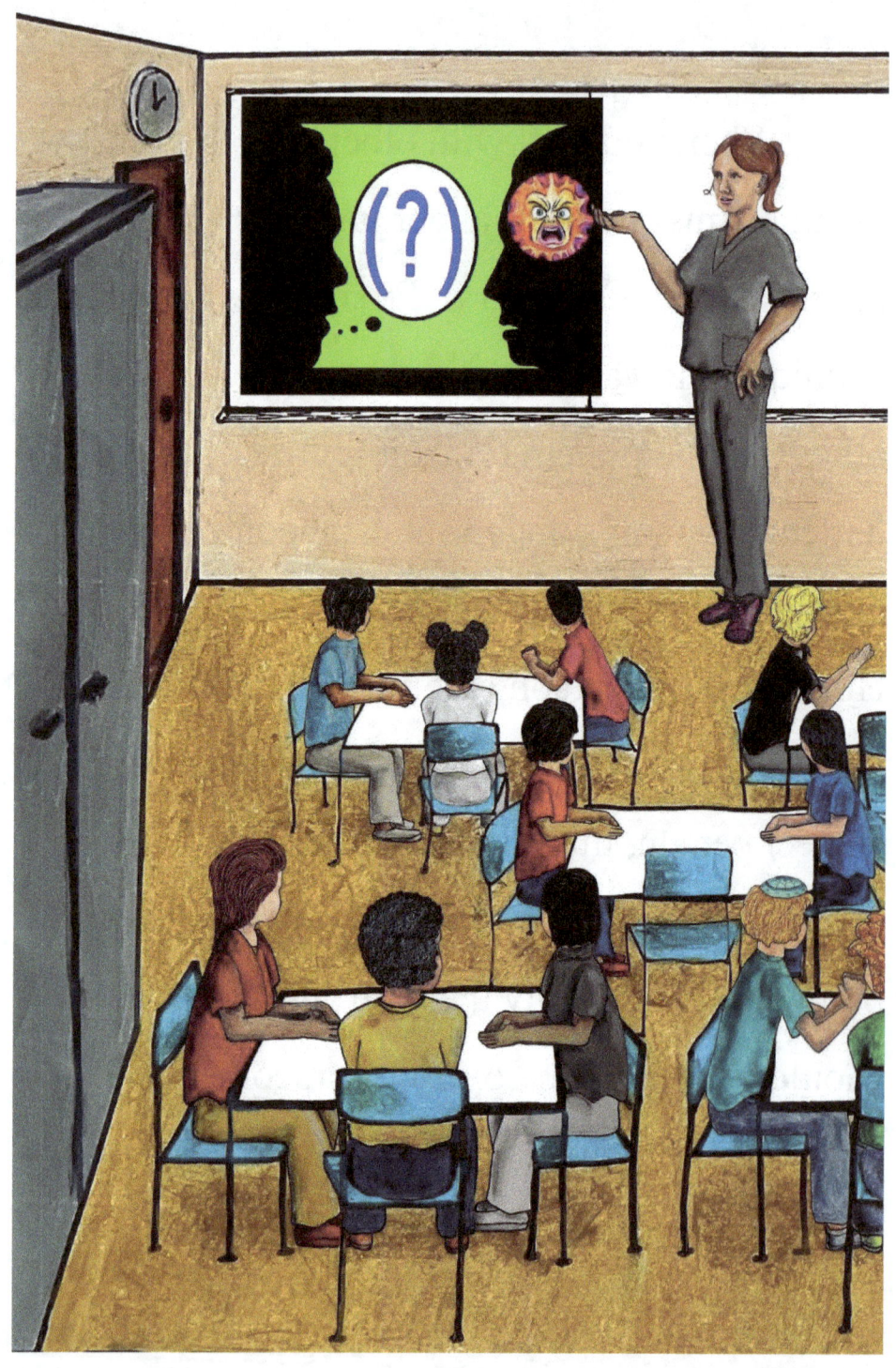

"When someone is angry, be a detective and ask for more details about the situation. Learn as much as you can, which will also help the other person develop an outside perspective of their anger so that they can withhold judgment if that is what is needed. Being a detective is a skill that must be practiced and strengthened."

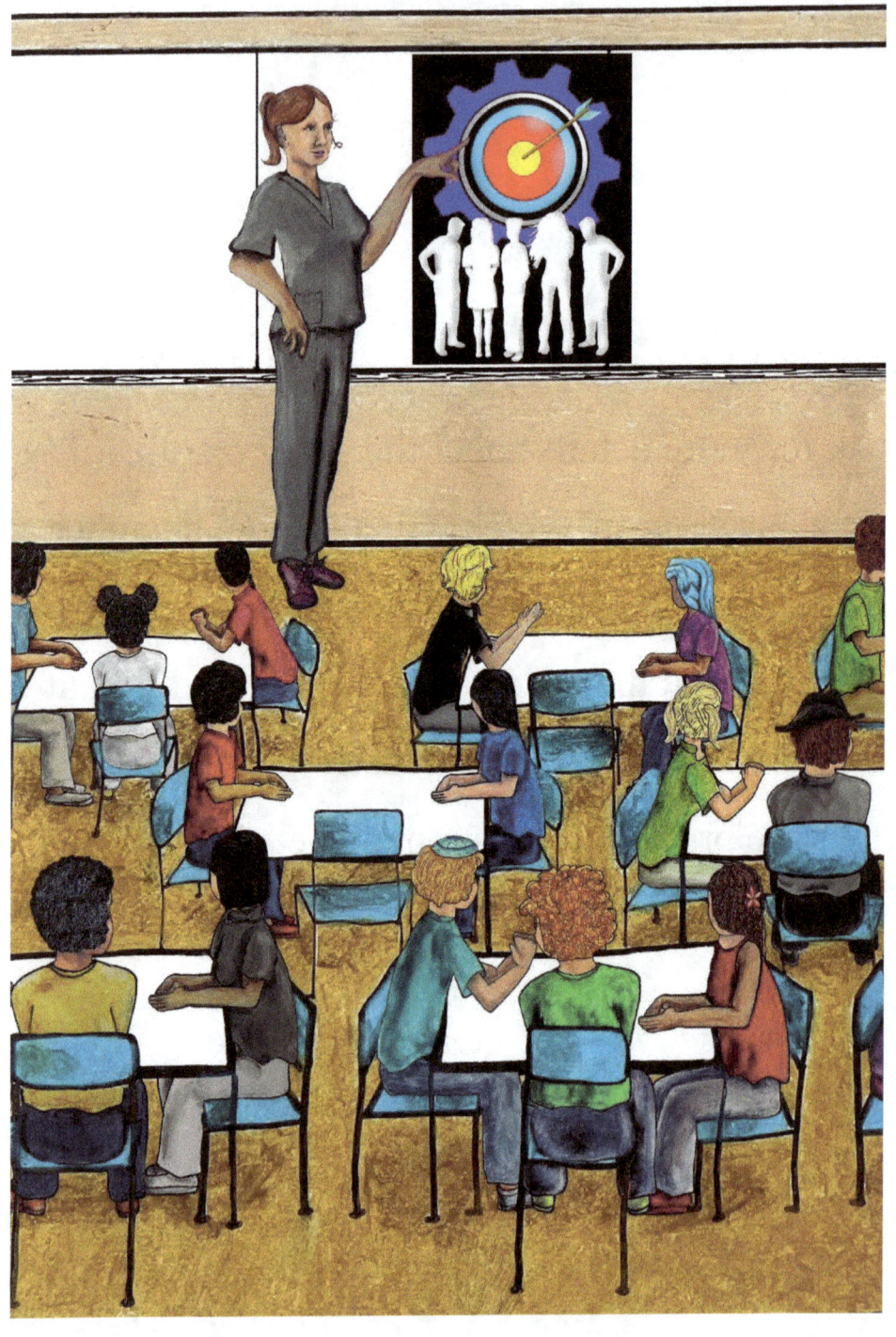

"If the anger is involving a business or team contribution of some kind, then consider having the team redesign goals together, so that anger is properly dealt with. The team becomes strengthened and develops stronger guidance with the help of each other."

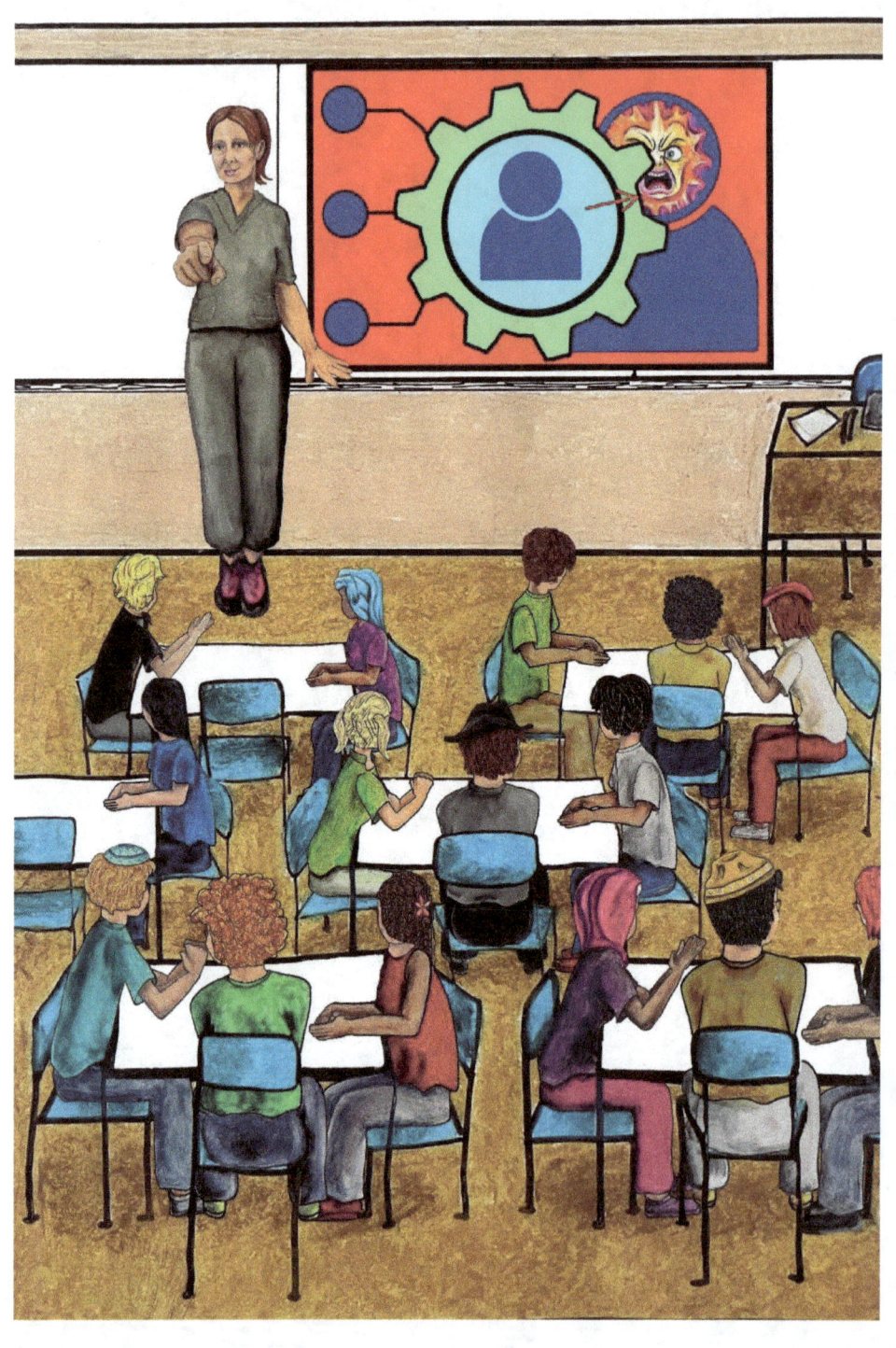

"Acknowledge any part that you may have played to make someone else angry."

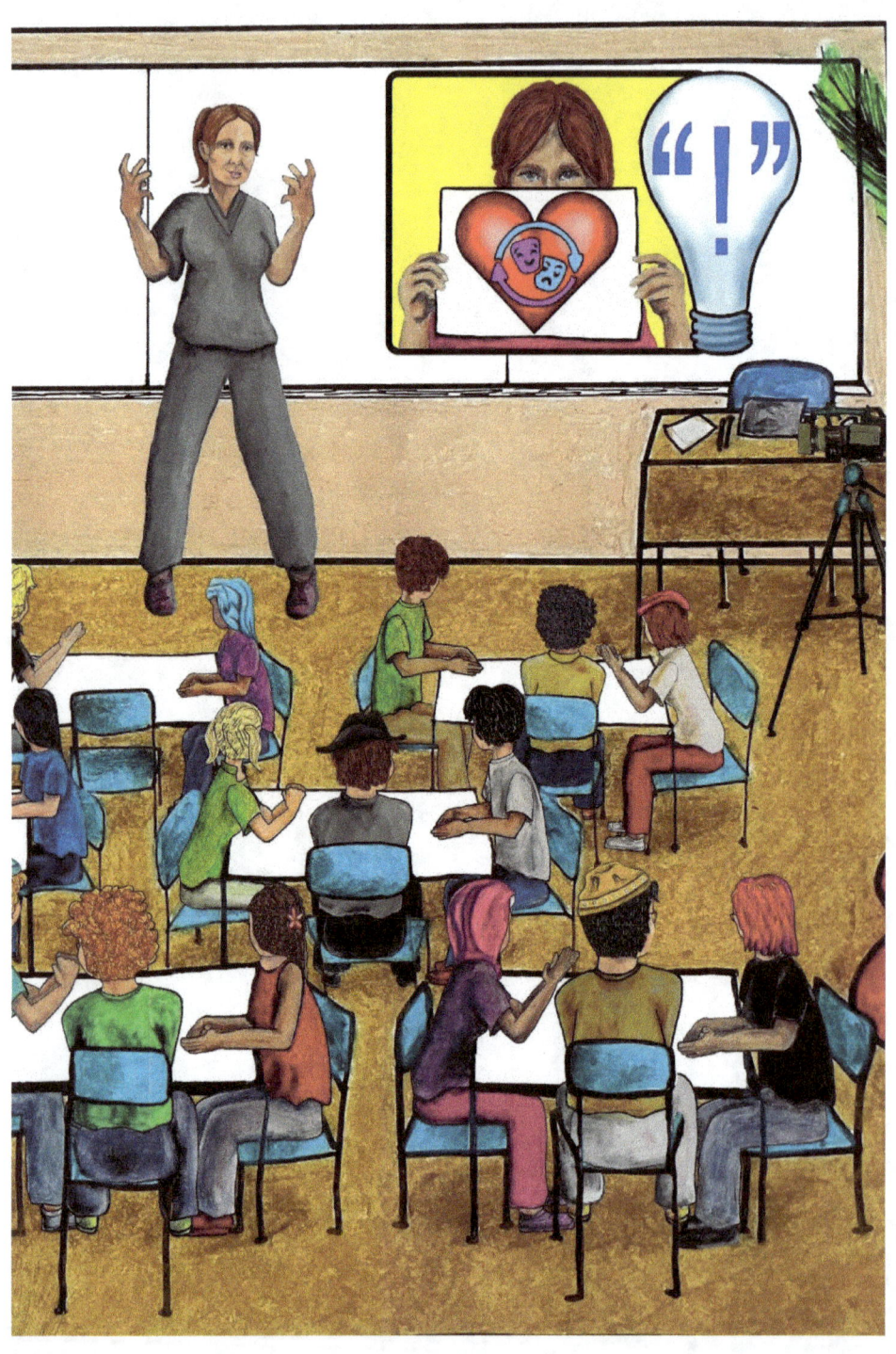

"It is good to feel the emotion of anger fully, but choose to make a good outcome with the anger. Get help managing your anger from anyone or anything that seems capable of providing an outside perspective. Finally, think about the disadvantages of acting on your anger. List out the possible negative consequences if you act on your anger."

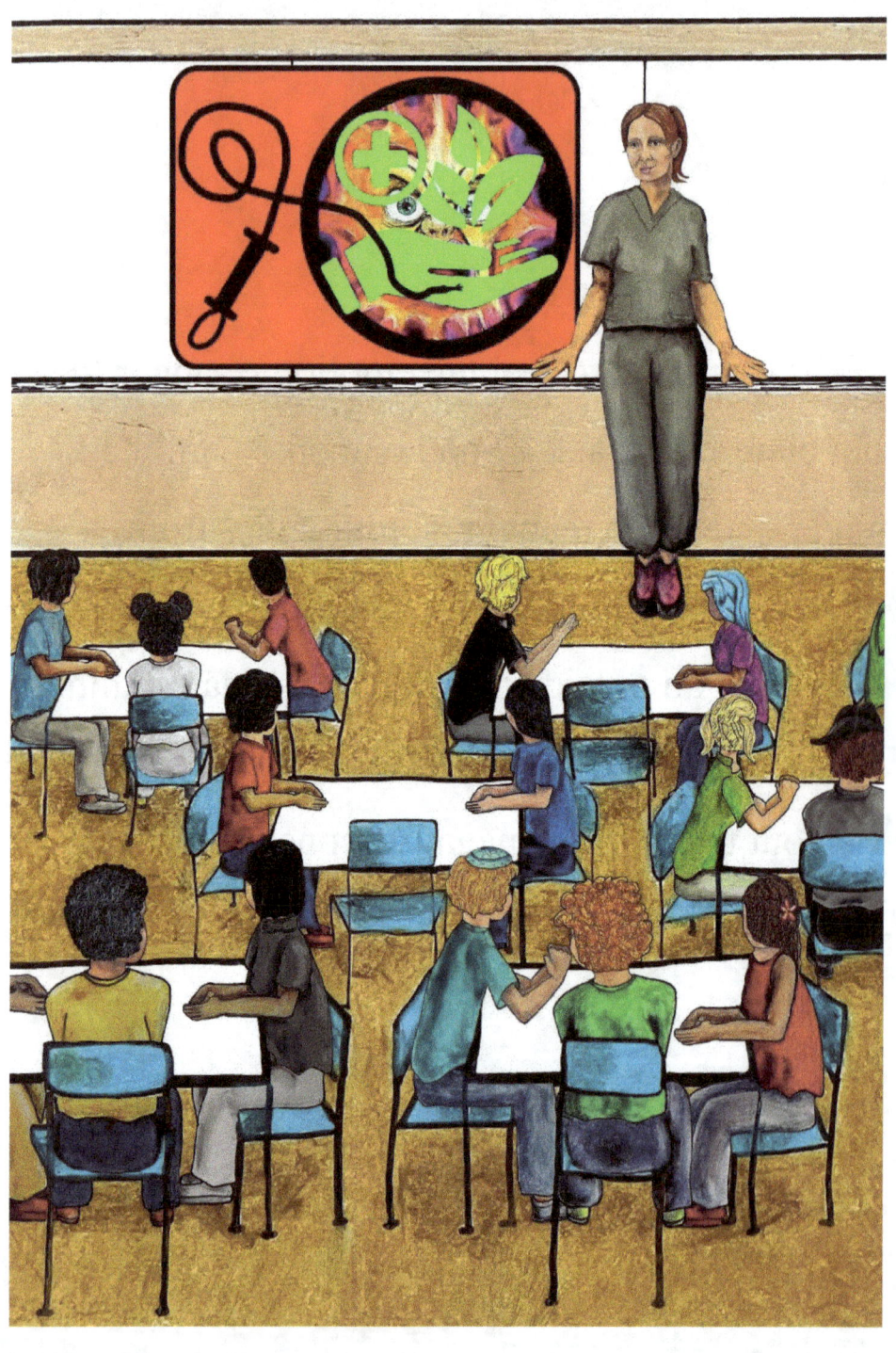

"Anger is a natural emotion like a wild horse in the wilderness. We must learn to tame it so that it can be useful for society. Just because a horse is wild doesn't mean it can never be ridden. Small incremental steps in managing anger may be needed, but eventually you will have tamed your anger and can use it as a creative force for the good of society."

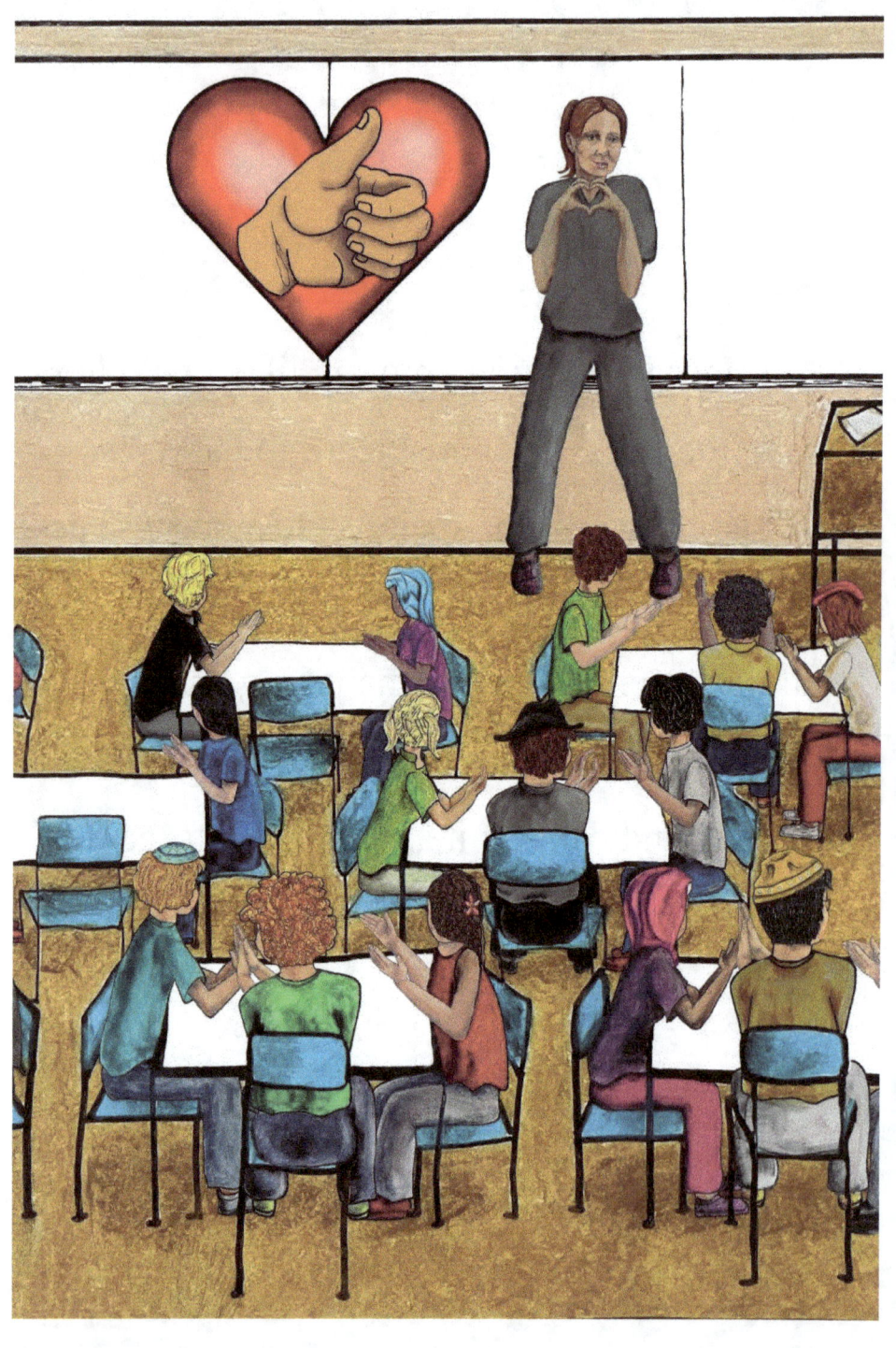

"This concludes my class on anger management. I hope you enjoyed it and learned many things to improve your mental well-being. I'll be around after class to answer any questions that you may have, but were afraid to ask in front of the group. Have a great rest of your day," says Nurse Dorothea. The class starts to clap, and many students say, "Thank you, Nurse Dorothea." Some come up to the nurse after the class is dismissed and give her a big hug, telling her how much she helped.

References

American Psychological Association. (2023). Control anger before it controls you. Retrieved from: https://www.apa.org/topics/anger/control

Bregman, P. (2014). What to Do When Anger Takes Hold. Retrieved from: https://hbr.org/2014/10/what-to-do-when-anger-takes-hold

Chhaya, N. (2022). Managing Anger, Frustration, and Resentment on Your Team. Retrieved from: https://hbr.org/2022/02/managing-anger-frustration-and-resentment-on-your-team

Holland, K. (2019). How to Control Anger: 25

Tips to Help You Stay Calm. Retrieved from: https://www.healthline.com/health/mental-health/how-to-control-anger#1

Ineffable Living. (n.d.) Top 14 CBT Anger Management Exercises (+FREE Anger Management Worksheets). Retrieved from: https://ineffableliving.com/manage-your-anger/

Mayo Clinic Staff. (2024). Anger management: 10 tips to tame your temper. Retrieved from: https://www.mayoclinic.org/healthy-lifestyle/adult-health/in-depth/anger-management/art-20045434

Mental Health America. (n.d.). 10 Healthy Ways to Release Rage. Retrieved from:

https://www.mhanational.org/10-healthy-ways-release-rage

Mental Health America. (n.d.). 18 Ways to Cope with Frustration. Retrieved from: https://www.mhanational.org/18-ways-cope-frustration

Morin, A. (2023). 11 Anger Management Strategies to Help You Calm Down. Retrieved from: https://www.verywellmind.com/anger-management-strategies-4178870

Sutton, J. (2021). Anger Management for Teens: Helpful Worksheets & Resources. Retrieved from: https://positivepsychology.com/anger-management-for-teens/

About the Illustrator

Lindsay acquired her BFA from Columbus College of Art and Design. She was a self-employed metal artist beginning in 1985 and was part of the American Arts and crafts movement of the late 80's and early 90's with an art piece on permanent collection at the White House and the governor's mansion in Ohio. The majority of the works she sold then were done in metal, either soldered or welded. During that time, she spent 5 years serving on the board of Ohio Designer Craftsmen and networked part of her business through them. She sold many of her works through art galleries across the USA and Japan. She did many individual commissions and was also commissioned to do giftware design through Bath and Body Works, i.e., the Limited, in the year 2000.

In 2008, Lindsay went back to college to acquire another degree so she could try her hand at teaching high school art. She acquired a M.Ed. from U of A. She taught art at 6 different schools in AZ before retiring in 2022. In her last 4 years, she taught: Art 1, Advanced Art, AP Art, Ceramics, Advanced Ceramics, and Photography I, II, III, and IV (which was also producing the school's yearbook). Several of her students were recipients of HAA Art scholarships. During her first year of teaching at public schools, she taught Graphic Design. All this time, she enjoyed making art with her students and building her illustration, drawing, and painting skills.

During those teaching years she still accomplished a few commissions of steel sculptures. It started with the first commission from Norton Abrasives of creating the company's mascot. It was a larger-than-life French bulldog named Cooper. Cooper resides at the company's US headquarters in Brownsville TX. The mascot had long lines during one trade show of people wanting to take selfies with it. It was a hit and resulted in a personal commission for a couple in Los Angeles of another bulldog named Sebastian.

When Lindsay retired in 2022, she worked with an old friend in Ohio who is an author and performer on a children's book. All the illustrations in the book including the cover were created by Lindsay. The book is for 0-8 year old children and is called "Sleep Little Raven".

Lindsay has kept a blog since 2008 showing the progress of her works at www.curlycu.com.

In Lindsay's words:
"Making art is like breathing; it is a must for my own survival and sanity."

About the Author

Michael is married to Perla in Tucson, AZ. Michael served in the US Air Force between 2002 and 2010 as an Electronic Warfare Officer on the EC-130H Compass Call and deployed 6 times in the Global War on Terror. Michael then served 8 years as an Army Wounded Warrior Advocate. Michael used his GI bill to go to nursing school and works as an RN at an inpatient psychiatric hospital in Tucson, AZ. Michael enjoys listening to Beethoven and reading a lot of news.

Michael's college education:

B.A. in Psychology from Auburn University,

B.S. in Biology from the University of Alabama at Birmingham,

M.S. in Management from Troy University,

Master in Health Administration from the University of Phoenix,

M.S. from the University of Arizona through the accelerated Master's Entry to the Profession of Nursing program

Other Books by Dow Creative Enterprises®

For info about other titles in the series, visit www.NurseDorothea.com

Visit www.DowCreativeEnterprises.com for more information about DCE

www.ingramcontent.com/pod-product-compliance
Lightning Source LLC
Chambersburg PA
CBHW052339230426
43664CB00041B/2375